Happy
Healthy
...Dead

Happy Healthy ...Dead

*Why What You Think You Know
About Aging Is Wrong and
How To Get It Right*

NOELLE C. NELSON

ISBN-13: 978-1517008970

ISBN-10: 1517008972

Media inquiries and contact:

Diane Rumbaugh

Rumbaugh Public Relations

diane@rumbaughpr.com

Cover art by Damonza.com

Formatting by Dazmonza.com

Inspiration for the book title from Abraham-Hicks, with thanks.

CONTENTS

Part I: What You Need to Know

Chapter One: Meet The Real Un-Dead: Happy Healthy Centenarians 3

Chapter Two: What You Think Is What You Live 13

Chapter Three: For Whom the Stress Tolls 19

Chapter Four: The Fix. 27

Chapter Five: What Makes Appreciation So Special? 33

Chapter Six: Hocus Pocus, the Magic of Focus 41

Part II: What You Need to Do

1. Step Away From the Comparison Game: Be Grateful to Be You! 55

2. *The Lion King* and *Aladdin* Get the Best of a Laguardia Situation. 59

3. Shape Your Life Up: Tell Yourself the (Desired) Truth . . 63

4. Turn "Yeah, But" on Its Head 67

5. Getting Your Nursing-Home-Phobic Spouse to Help With Mom 71

6. Smile! It's Good for Your Health 75

7. What Improv Theatre Taught Me About "Yes, and" 79

8. Become an Optimist In Three Easy Steps 83

9. Terrified of Getting Older 87

10. I Should Have Married a Mind Reader!. 89

11. Put Grit In Your Personal Goals 93

12. My Way or the Highway. Really?! 97

13. Taking Those Car Keys Away: With or Without Drama? . 101

14. Want Success? Focus on What Works 105

15. Tip Your Marital Scales Into Joy 109

16. Waste Not, Want Not 113

17. Be Truly Human: Practice Random Acts of Kindness. 115

18. A Non-Waste of Time Team-Building Exercise Worth Trying At Home 119

19. Living In "Can't Do/Don't Have" Mode? Try Living In "Can Do" Mode 123

20. What I Learned From Yucky Fish 127

21. Want More Life Satisfaction? Supercharge Your Work . 129

22. Why Me? Every Woman's Lament 133

23. Is It Your Mood or Your Attitude? 137

24. How to Make Worry Your Friend (!) 141

25. Let Go or Get Dragged 145

26. Attitude of Gratitude? (Yeah, Right...) 149

27. Are You Listening Competitively? Or Listening to Learn? . 153

28. Collateral Benefits: Be Good to Your Mate, It's Good for Your Health 157

29. Choose Your Thought Reps Wisely 161

30. Celebrate Your Life With Love on Valentine's Day. . . 165

31. Fill Your Life With Happiness: Make It Meaningful . 169

32. The "Just One" Secret to Fitness (Or Anything Else) . 173

33. Appreciate Your Obnoxious Crazy Relatives? Sure! Why Not? 177

34. Will Boredom Steal Your Love Away? 181

35. Anger: Release First, Appreciate Second 185

36. Ditch the "Have-to's" and Get to the (Way More Fun) "Want-to's" 189

37. Women Complain, Men Leave 193

38. Don't Leave Yourself Out of Thanksgiving Gratitude . 197

LAST WORDS 201

REFERENCES. 203

RESOURCES. 211

ABOUT THE AUTHOR. 215

PART I

What You Need to Know

CHAPTER ONE

Meet The Real Un-Dead: Happy Healthy Centenarians

"Tell me, what is it you plan to do with your one wild and precious life?"

Mary Oliver

I travel a great deal for work. One day I was on a plane, the flight attendant had gone through her safety-procedures routine, including the usual "airplane-mode only during take-off" announcement. The young man next to me, well ensconced in his window-seat and ear-buds, continued to text. I figured perhaps he hadn't heard the announcement, so as the attendants closed the doors, I leaned towards him and said, "We're taking off. You need to put your phone in airplane mode." He barely glanced at me, and continued to click away. The plane started down the runway. I repeated myself, "Uh, hello! You need to switch to airplane mode. Your phone's signal could interfere with the pilot's radio frequencies. It's not safe."

The young man shot me a disdainful look and said, "What would you know? You're ooold." That stopped me cold. Then I replied, "If you're lucky, if you're very, very lucky, you'll get to be old like me." Mind you, I hadn't yet turned 60.

That is where the problem lies. Most of us want to live a long life, but very few of us want to actually get old. Or as my young friend on the plane said, "ooold."

I remember my grandmothers—both my grandmothers, for that matter—and both of them, by their late 50s, were considered old. They were expected to do no more than sit quietly, placid, while the world moved around them, a role they accepted without protest. My maternal grandmother would crochet little dresses for our dolls. My dad's mom would "fuss" as my mother put it. She'd squint through her reading glasses, looking for something to dust or re-arrange, getting up slowly every so often to do so. They were to be spared any hard work or aggravation. "Don't bother your grandmother!" was the most frequent refrain we children heard during family get-togethers.

That's changed, have you noticed? 60 may not be the new 40, and who knows if 70 is the new 50, but one thing is for sure: we're living longer, and most of us are refusing the sedentary veg-til-you-die approach to our later years.

A long happy, healthy life. That's what we're aiming for, aren't we? With yogurt and yoga, and brain games. I take ballet and fully expect to be dancing on YouTube at 90. Why not? I'll call it, "The wrinkled ballerina takes the floor."

And yet, when people are asked, "Have you planned for retirement?" or "What are your concerns for your future after retirement?" just about everyone says, "How will I be able to pay all those health costs?" As if the great majority of us expect to spend all those years after retirement in a continually progressive debilitated state, finally ending up in a hospital, sprouting tubes: the inevitable finale to that ever-more-painful lingering decline towards death.

How utterly and totally depressing! Granted, no one gets out of here alive, but let's at least *live* until it's time to die. Let our emphasis be on how happy we can make ourselves and our lives, such that our focus is on "happy, healthy" with "dead" being but a final punctuation mark.

Our mental pictures of anyone over 75 are pathetic. And over 80, 90, 100—even worse. Television is rife with ads promoting cures or solace for the infirmities that we are all supposedly doomed to as we age: Alzheimer's, incontinence, diabetic neuralgia, chronic pain and ill health, the need for wheelchairs, walkers. We're told that without an electronic device slung around our necks to summon help, we'll crumple to the ground from a heart attack and die there: wretched, alone and in agony!

It's no wonder that no one wants to grow old, that old age scares the heck out of us. And yet, as I told the young man in the plane, we who live long lives are the lucky ones! The survivors, those who made it, so to speak, past the perilous 20s, ambitious 30s and 40s, the questioning 50s and beyond.

This is not to say that there aren't some older individuals who suffer from Alzheimer's, severe cognitive impairment, arthritic joints, broken hips and a whole host of other afflictions, but there are far more individuals in their 10s, 20s, 30s and 40s who are dealing with a variety of disorders such as cancer, rheumatoid arthritis, deformed or amputated limbs, an astonishing array of injuries from various accidents, and cognitive issues of all kinds.

The difference is that we don't automatically assign an entire class of individuals to certain misery just by virtue of their age—except for the elderly. Past the age of 65, and certainly by the time you hit 75, pretty much everyone expects you to need a walker, be diabetic, and have heart issues.

This, despite the fact that according to the 2011 US Census Bureau's report, only 3.1 percent of the total population 65 years and over live in a nursing home.[1]

And again, despite the fact that well-known figures such as:

Clint Eastwood, at 84, directed the award-winning *American Sniper* and *Jersey Boys* movies, both released in 2014.

Angela Lansbury, at 89, toured England and the United States in 2014, in the title role of Noel Coward's *Blithe Spirit*—for which she had received a Tony in 2009.

Dick Van Dyke, at 88, completed work on *Night at the Museum: Secret of the Tomb* in 2014, and starred in a music video for folk music band Dustbowl Revival in 2015—at 89.

Betty White, at 89 and 90, received the 2011 and 2012 Screen Actors Guild awards for Outstanding Performance by a Female Actor in a Comedy Series (*Hot in Cleveland*), and whose Great American Country special *Betty White's Smartest Animals in America* aired on her birthday in January 2015—at 93.

Norman Lear, at 93, still fulfilling his bucket list. Latest on the agenda? He lip-synched a song by Paul Hipp in a funny, touching YouTube salute to his 93rd birthday.[2] Lear, best known for his TV producer success (*All in the Family*, *The Jeffersons*, *Maude* among others), continues to pursue his long standing passion—the promotion of active and thoughtful American citizenship.

Lest you think you have to be in show business to live a long, happy, productive life, there's Henry Kissinger. In 2014 at 91, Kissinger published his most recent of over a dozen books on politics and international relations, *World Order* (New York, Penguin Press), and continues to be active in a number of groups and think tanks concerned with foreign relations, among other activities.

Then there are those individuals who are not so well known:

Phyllis Sues celebrated her 92nd birthday in 2015 by performing an amazing tango which was uploaded to YouTube amid great acclaim. Considering that Sues began taking tango (and trapeze) at 80, that's quite something. Oh, and did I mention she learned Italian and French in her 70s?[3]

BKS Iyengar, a master teacher, was photographed at 95 doing his yoga stances. He was one of the foremost names in yoga, training such luminaries as violinist Yehudi Menuhin, Madonna and the Queen of Belgium. His achievement is all the more astonishing given that he was born in 1918 during an influenza epidemic and was a weak, malnourished child whose many illnesses included malaria, tuberculosis and typhoid.[4]

Ed Robles, 88, is a World War II veteran, who as of 2015 has been a volunteer for about 16 years with the Retired Senior Volunteer Patrol, patrolling the streets of San Diego, California in a police car, along with his senior patrol buddy, a pilot who served in the Vietnam War.[5] San Diego's oldest patrol volunteer was 92.

Robles is not the only senior helping out local police. The Douglas Wyoming Police Department's oldest volunteer is a woman in her 90s. The Toledo Ohio Police Department says that the peak age for volunteers seems to be 87. Their most senior volunteer in 2015 was 85.

What about all those centenarians?

In the 2010 U.S. census, there were 53,364 centenarians, defined as people 100 years and over, a 5.8 percent increase from the 2000 census when there were 50,454 people who were at least 100 years old. That means that of the total population in 2010, 1 out of every 5,786 people was a centenarian.[6] Given those averages, it's likely that wherever you live, there are one or more centenarians living close by.

Healthy, happy centenarians defy the stereotype of decrepit old age. They are active and involved in life and living.

People such as:

Astrid Thoenig, who celebrated her 100th birthday by going to work, as she has for the last 30 years, at an insurance company in New Jersey. In her capacity as the office manager,

Thoenig answers phones, handles payroll and other financial records, and types up documents. In 2013 she was still on the job at 103, saying, "I don't think old and I don't feel old."[7]

New Zealander Bob Edwards, on the road (legally!) in 2013, driving around at age 105.[8]

Margaret Dunning, well known on the classic car circuit, and a loving restorer of classic cars— doing many of the minor restoration and repairs herself—drove one of her fine automobiles in the Woodward Dream Cruise in Detroit each August up into her centenarian years. At 102 in 2013 she was still changing her own oil.[9]

George Blevins, who has been bowling regularly for 93 years, won his most recent National Senior Games singles tournaments for the over 75 age group at age 100.[10]

Lillian Weber celebrated her 100th birthday in 2015 by surpassing her goal of sewing 1,000 dresses for needy children—she sewed 1,051, all handmade, all personalized.[11]

John W. Donnelly received yet another gold medal for winning the National Senior Games table tennis championship—at 100 years of age. Table tennis isn't his only passion. He married his wife Marian at 94, with whom he toured Europe at 99.[12]

Margaret Dell, who lived to 104, was interviewed extensively by *Time* when she was 96. In addition to being the designated driver for her seventy-something friends, she knitted baby booties, caps and blankets for family and friends, played tennis several times a week, and according to her daughter-in-law, had "a light in her eyes that is very alive, alert and interested."[13]

How do centenarians do that thing they do: live for so long, active and healthy? Is it their diet, exercise, weight management, their alcohol or smoke-free lifestyle?

No! Amazingly enough, some centenarians drink alcohol, others don't, some eat "healthy," others don't, some pay attention to their weight, others don't, some smoke, others don't, some exercise, others wouldn't dream of it.

Although this isn't a reason to cut loose on the bacon-fried-ice-cream and tequila shots and declare that couch-potato is the life for you (because all those behaviors do indeed negatively impact your short and long-term health*), what is abundantly clear is that centenarians pursue a variety of life-styles.

Some centenarians have downright intriguing habits to which they attribute their longevity. One 110 year old advocates drinking a can of beer a day. A 107 year old attributes her long life to drinking lots of coffee. A 109er says staying away from men will do it (you have to wonder what men are supposed to do). An Italian 115 year old advocates eating raw eggs. A 116 year old Japanese says "sunbathe," and a 117 year old says "eat sushi"![14]

The one thing—the only thing—that centenarians have in common is their positive attitude.

They aren't whiners. They are happy. They are optimistic. Above all, the "long-lived" appreciate the ordinary moments of everyday life.

You may think being happy, optimistic, positive and appreciative are nice ways to feel, pleasant ways to go about life, but they go far beyond momentary feel-goods. Happiness, optimism, positive attitude and appreciation have tremendous consequences for your physical well-being, for your longevity. They may be, in fact, the missing link between you today, and a happy, healthy you tomorrow—and tomorrow, and tomorrow.

With that, let's look at just how that happens, starting with your body.

This book is not meant to replace what you and/or your health care providers have decided is the best course of action for your physical, mental and emotional well-being, but rather to enhance and support what you are already doing to assure your happy, healthy longevity.

CHAPTER TWO

What You Think Is What You Live

"The mind is everything. What you think you become."

Buddha

It's obvious that what we eat, ingest, smoke or snort has an impact on our bodies. It's equally obvious that subjecting our bodies to severe weather, slamming into doors, blunt objects, or falling down stairs also has an impact on our bodies. What we don't pause to consider is how what we think and the emotions we feel impact our bodies.

It turns out that what you think and feel has far greater impact on your physical well-being, and—more to the point of this discussion—on your happy, healthy longevity than you may realize. Sometimes, even more impact than whatever you may be doing physically.

Stick with me, all will be revealed. First, some science.

Your thoughts and your feelings result in the release of particular chemicals from your brain, and from certain cells in your body. These chemicals, called neuropeptides, act like messengers, bringing information about your thoughts and feelings to specific receptor sites on your cells. These receptor sites, upon receiving this mental and emotional information, are now equipped to tell your cells how to respond, what to do.

Every single one of the major systems in your body—your nervous system, your hormonal system, your gastrointestinal system, your immune system, your cardiovascular system—all of your bodily systems are set up to communicate with one another.

Every second, a massive information exchange is occurring in your body, via the neuropeptides and their corresponding receptor sites, linking all of your bodily systems and your mind. Your body and your mind are not separate, not at all.

Your thoughts and emotions are in fact cellular signals that are involved in the process of translating information into physical reality. The condition of your body and how you feel is to a surprisingly large degree a direct biochemical result of what you think and what you feel.

This close interaction between thought, emotion, and bodily systems explains why recent widows are twice as likely to develop breast cancer, and why individuals who suffer from chronic depression are four times more likely to get sick.[1] It also explains the results of a study that observed the health of 255 medical students for 25 years. Those who were the most hostile had five times greater occurrence of coronary heart disease than those who were not hostile.[2]

That's the downside. Negative thoughts and feelings have an impact on your physical being. However, there is an opposite and equally powerful upside, perhaps best exemplified in the classic 1979 study by a group of Harvard psychologists, spearheaded by Ellen Langer, PhD.[3]

The psychologists selected a group of healthy men, aged seventy-five or older, who then spent a week at a retreat. The retreat was decorated in keeping with the styles, reading materials and music of 1959, the year in which these men would have been in their mid-fifties.

- The men were not allowed to talk about anything that had happened since 1959, and were to talk in the present tense about their families, careers, and lives as if it were actually 1959.

- They discussed the topics of the day—circa 1959 and before—and viewed movies from that era.

- They were given photo identification of themselves at their 1959 ages, and learned to refer to each other by looking at those pictures.

- The men were treated as if they had the intelligence and independence of younger men, and given complex instructions to follow about their daily routine, even though in their regular lives many of these men were dependent on younger family members to perform daily tasks for them.

- The men were asked their opinions on various matters in a respectful way, and those opinions were actually listened to—something that almost never happened in their regular lives.

- In other words, the men were appreciated. Who they were and what they had to say was valued. Their ability and intelligence were appreciated in the same way they had been when they were twenty years younger.

The physical results on these men after this brief week-long retreat in which they were valued, appreciated, and experienced positive states of being, are nothing short of amazing.

- Impartial judges who examined photographs of the men before and after the retreat observed that the men looked visibly younger after the retreat by an average of three years.

- People's fingers tend to shorten with age, yet the men's fingers were found to have lengthened after this brief experiment.

- Their joints became more flexible.

- Their posture began to straighten, resembling more the posture they had when they were younger.

- Their muscle strength improved, their hearing improved and their eyesight improved.

- Not only that, but over half of the "1959ers" scored

higher on IQ tests after the retreat, even though intelligence is usually considered to be unchangeable once you're an adult.

Other, more recent studies, such as research done at Duke University, reported that in the 866 heart patients the researchers observed, those who routinely felt more positive emotions had a 20 percent greater likelihood of being alive 11 years later than the heart patients who usually experienced more negative emotions.[4]

Not only that, but a Johns Hopkins study reported that even in adults at risk of heart disease due to their family history, a positive outlook offered the strongest known protection against heart disease—as well as or even better than maintaining an appropriate diet, exercise regimen or body weight.[5]

You are in charge of what you think. And what you think impacts how your body responds. You can choose thoughts that support positive emotions, just as you can choose thoughts that support negative emotions.

In the land of happy, healthy longevity, positive emotions rule. No, this isn't some cutesy New Age wishful thinking. It's research and science-based. So before we move on to how to access those positive emotions, which thoughts are most effective and why, we'll take a deeper look at what scientists have to say about the impact that what you think and what you feel has on your health and longevity.

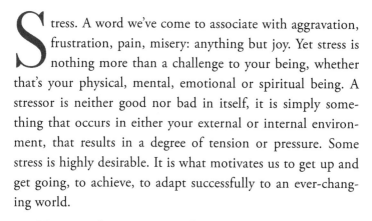

CHAPTER THREE

For Whom the Stress Tolls

"Stress is an ignorant state. It believes that everything is an emergency."

Natalie Goldberg

Stress. A word we've come to associate with aggravation, frustration, pain, misery: anything but joy. Yet stress is nothing more than a challenge to your being, whether that's your physical, mental, emotional or spiritual being. A stressor is neither good nor bad in itself, it is simply something that occurs in either your external or internal environment, that results in a degree of tension or pressure. Some stress is highly desirable. It is what motivates us to get up and get going, to achieve, to adapt successfully to an ever-changing world.

However, the stress most of us think of isn't the positive

motivating variety. It's the stress of too many responsibilities and obligations, not enough money/health/work/love/time, of accidents and crises involving ourselves or loved ones, disastrous relationships, and so on. The hardships of life. Yet, what kills us isn't the stress itself, it's our response to stress. It's what we think and how we feel about the stressor that damages our health and shortens our lives.

For example, there you are minding your own business, and your boss says, "Could I see you for a moment in my office, please?" If your thoughts are along the lines of, "What did I do wrong now? Did I do/say something horribly inappropriate? Am I about to get fired?" you'll trigger fearful emotions, all centered around, "How am I going to survive this? Am I going to survive this?" Your body follows your lead, faithful servant that it is, with the classic "flight or fight" response, preparing you to survive what you've defined as a potentially life-threatening crisis.

Now let's say that to top it off, your boss says, "On second thought, I've got some other things to take care of. Come see me first thing tomorrow." Not only can you not run and hide (flight), nor can you duke it out verbally with your boss (fight), but now you have to wait until the next day, which gives you a whole afternoon, evening, night and morning through which you maintain an elevated inflammatory response throughout your body. That hyper-alert "flight or fight" response, which although a normal and natural part of your body's ability to protect itself via your immune system, was never meant to stay in "on" mode. You keep that up a day, a week, a month, a year, and you're damaging your health and potential longevity.

A high stress response to everyday situations can lead to

chronic inflammation. Chronic inflammation occurs through-out your body when a stressor triggers your immune system, and instead of turning itself off, your immune system con-tinues to deliver immune cells that interfere with your body's healthy tissues. What started out as a good, protective immune system function becomes a destructive, harmful one.

Chronic inflammation contributes significantly to health problems such as cancer, heart disease, obesity, and more specifically, age-related conditions such as frailty and cogni-tive decline.

Researchers at Penn State have found that people who remain calm or cheerful in the face of ordinary stressors have a lower risk of inflammation. According to the study's primary author, Dr. Nancy Sin, "A person's frequency of stress may be less related to inflammation than responses to stress. It is how a person reacts to stress that is important...Positive emotions, and how they can help people in the event of stress, have really been overlooked."[1]

Imagine that instead of your habitual irritation, fear or anger, you reacted to your boss's "Could I see you for a moment in my office, please?" with thoughts such as, "Huh, I wonder what's up?" "Oh good, maybe I'll get a chance to talk with the boss about my new idea." When you're not thinking and feeling fear, the same "Come to my office please" from your boss has virtually no impact on your body. That's how powerful our thoughts and feelings are. That's the biochemis-try linking them.

But there's more. Even the conservative Centers for Disease Control and Prevention (CDC) states that 85 percent of all diseases have an emotional element. [2] When you think and feel anger, fear, resentment or despair, you put your health and longevity at risk, even beyond the already discussed heightened inflammatory response.

Your heart, for example, is a highly emotionally responsive organ. When you are positive, cheerful and content, your heart beats with a calm, smooth, steady rhythm. It can thus accomplish its main function well, which is to pump blood throughout your body, so that your cells receive the oxygen and nutrients they need to produce energy, even as carbon dioxide and other wastes are removed. It's an amazingly well-orchestrated system that assures your well-being without your conscious thought or interference.[3]

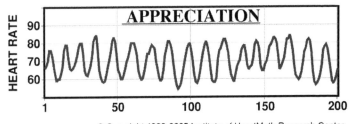

© Copyright 1998-2005 Institute of HeartMath Research Center

However, when you are in the grip of anger, fear, or other powerful negative thoughts and feelings, your heart rate becomes chaotic, irregular, and unpredictable, which means it no longer pumps blood in an orderly manner to your cells. Such a disordered heart rhythm has consequences, such as high blood pressure, which in turn contributes to hardening of the arteries, stroke, kidney disease, and even to the development of heart failure. All of which, if they don't end up contributing to your demise, certainly can prematurely age you.[4]

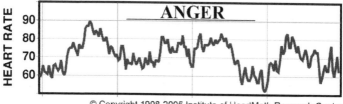

© Copyright 1998-2005 Institute of HeartMath Research Center

You think your heart is responsive? Try your brain!

Your brain requires blood flowing to it in order to function. Guess what determines, to a large degree, the pattern of how blood flows—or doesn't—to various parts of your brain? Your thoughts, once again, what you think and feel. The extensive brain-study research done by scientists such as Dr. Daniel Amen and Dr. M.S. George has demonstrated that depending on what you are thinking and feeling, parts of your brain are either turned on, or turned off, which in turn has everything to do with how your mind works, and how you behave.[5]

When you are experiencing positive thoughts and feelings—in particular, appreciation—blood is flowing as it should throughout your brain, so that you can function at your very best. You have no trouble focusing your thoughts. Your memory is right there. You are motivated and energized. Your coordination is solid. You don't get readily tweaked. You tolerate the bumps and hurdles of life more easily. You are in a very good place.

Your Brain On Appreciation

(SPECT study measuring blood flow—shown as black patches—to the brain: underside view of the brain)

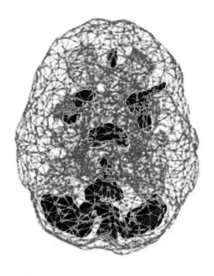

When you are experiencing negative thoughts and feelings, however, the exact opposite is happening. The blood flow to your cerebellum, which controls integrated movement, is greatly diminished. In addition, your left temporal lobe, which keeps you on an even keel, doesn't receive enough blood flow. The upshot is, you become klutzy and your coordination is impaired. You become emotionally unstable, and get anxious or fearful for no apparent reason. You don't think straight and can't seem to remember things. You're quicker to get frustrated, angry and act out.[6]

Your Brain On Anger

*(SPECT study measuring blood flow—shown as black patches—
to the brain: underside view of the brain)*

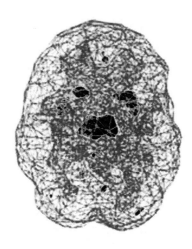

None of which is conducive to happy, healthy longevity! If you're uncoordinated, you're more likely to fall, you may become accident-prone, susceptible to injury. If you're anxious or fearful, you inadvertently trigger your flight-or-fight response, with the unfortunate consequence of chronic inflammation. Repeated anger and frustration only damage your immune system further. If you can't think straight and are always forgetting things, you won't be able to take good care of yourself. Not a pretty picture.

Fortunately, there is a solution, what I think of as "The Fix."

CHAPTER FOUR

The Fix

"Misery has enough company. Dare to be happy."

Volkswagen ad

Get out your Sherlock Holmes deerstalker cap and meerschaum pipe—or your Batman cape, whatever floats your boat. In a word, we're going sleuthing.

Who lives long? What is it the happy, healthy long-lived do that others don't?

1. They are happy

Well, that's kind of "duh," but here's the science backing it up.

In the classic "Nun Study," researchers analyzed autobiographies from 180 Catholic nuns, written when the nuns were in their early 20s, and then looked at the survival rate of the nuns between the ages of 75 and 95. The nuns who expressed gratitude, happiness, and positive emotions lived as much as *ten years longer* than those expressing fewer positive emotions. The study's primary author, David A. Snowdon PhD, stated that these findings agreed with "... other studies that have shown that people who rated more positive on personality tests were more likely to live longer than those who were more pessimistic... It feels good to be happy and hopeful. It's an enjoyable state that produces very little stress, and the body thrives in those conditions."[1]

In a 2011 study, researchers at University College, London, gauged the happiness levels of people ages 52 to 79 by monitoring their feelings several times over a day. Then, five years later, the researchers examined how many of those people had died. The result? Older people who are happy have a *35 percent lower risk of dying* over a five-year period than unhappy people. Even after the researchers controlled for medical conditions including cancer and diabetes, and health risks such as smoking, being happy was *still* linked with living longer. As noted by one of the study's foremost researchers, Professor Andrew Steptoe, "I was a bit surprised that the happiness effect was so strong even among people who had chronic diseases."[2]

2. They are grateful

Researcher and professor Robert Emmons believes strongly in the tremendous value of gratitude—being thankful for the good things we've received—and its connection to helping people cope with stress, a primary cause of chronic inflammation.[3] Highly grateful people have stronger immune systems, are sick less often, have lower blood pressure, and experience less depression and anxiety, all of which are strongly linked to greater longevity.[4]

Gratitude supports cardiovascular health as well as a healthy immune system, according to a study published in the American Journal of Cardiology. Once again, researchers found that cultivating gratitude significantly reduces stress, which in turn boosts immune function and overall health, both of which contribute to longevity.[5]

By how much does gratitude reduce stress? A paper released by the John Templeton Foundation shows that grateful people have 10 percent fewer stress-related illnesses and 12 percent lower blood pressure. Not only that, but grateful people tend to live up to *seven years longer* than average.[6]

Research out of UC Berkeley found that, regardless of life circumstances, grateful people are more satisfied with their lives than people who aren't grateful.[7] The relationship of life satisfaction to longevity is significant. A study published in *Psychological Science* in June 2015 followed 4,500 participants, all older than 50 years of age, over a period of nine years. Those whose satisfaction with their life overall was high had a "risk of mortality" (likelihood of death) *reduced by 18 percent*. Simply put, the more satisfied people are with their lives, the longer they live. This finding held true for people who had high levels of life satisfaction regardless of how their life satisfaction may have varied over time.[8]

3. They are optimistic

Optimists—characterized by their hopeful and confident attitude about the future—thrive. Their immune function is better, as evidenced from a number of studies. One study observed the immune systems of healthy first year law students, all under the mega-stress of law school. According to Lisa Aspinwall, PhD, psychology professor at the University of Utah, it was found that by mid-term, optimistic students had stronger immune systems (as measured by a certain class of protective blood cells) than those students characterized as pessimistic.[9]

In addition, Dr. Martin Seligman's extensive review of the research on optimists shows that optimists not only do better at work, school and sports, they recover from setbacks more quickly, and are less likely to become depressed. They are happier, calmer and generally at peace with themselves and life. Significantly, the research shows that optimists tend to be healthier, live longer, and age well.[10]

A Mayo Clinic study that followed more than 800 people for 30 years, once again showed that optimists live longer than pessimists. Even after factoring age and sex into the results, the researchers found that the optimistic group's actual survival rate was significantly better than what their expected survival was. Unfortunately, those in the pessimistic group had a 19% increase in risk of death.[11]

A survey of over 51,000 ethnically diverse Americans between the ages of 45 and 84 showed that optimists have amazing heart health; they are twice as likely to be in ideal cardiovascular health as compared to pessimists.[12] Given that cardiovascular disease is, according to the CDC, the leading cause of death in the United States, a healthy heart is a significant contributor to longevity.[13]

4. They are appreciative

Appreciation and gratitude are often used interchangeably, but they are in fact quite different. Gratitude is giving thanks for something received, whereas appreciation is acknowledging the value of something—the positive meaning it has for you—whether it's something received or simply observed.

Appreciation of the ordinary experiences of life is a hallmark of the long-lived, even more so of those who've passed the century mark. In his remarkable study of 1,200 people over 100 years of age, Albert Rosenfeld found that centenarians were generally happy with their jobs, their families, and their religion. Nearly all expressed a strong will to live, and had few regrets. Most importantly, the centenarians had great appreciation for the simple experiences and pleasures of life.[14]

Similarly, Dr. Stephen P. Jewett's New York study of the healthy long-lived (87 and older) revealed that they enjoyed life, appreciating its simple pleasures, and were able to see beauty where others only found ugliness.[15]

Dr. Dean Ornish of the University of California Medical School best sums up the impact of appreciation on longevity: "Regarding appreciation, I am not aware of any other factor in medicine—not diet, not smoking, not exercise, not stress, not genetics, not drugs, not surgery—that has a greater positive impact on quality of life, incidence of disease, fitness, and prevention of premature death."[16]

That's it! Appreciation is the key. It is what unlocks your ability to be happy, grateful and optimistic, which in turn results in an enhanced immune system, better cardiovascular health, and the various other factors which contribute to long-term well-being.

Here's how it works. When you appreciate, you think about the value something has for you, what it means to you. When something has meaning for you, when it matters to you, you can't help but be grateful for it; gratitude follows naturally on the heels of appreciation. When you appreciate something, and feel grateful for it, happiness ensues. And with that, you feel more hopeful about life and about the future, you are optimistic.

You've just set yourself up for a long, happy, healthy life. Great! But how do you make sense of all this? How do you translate it into the reality of *your* life?

CHAPTER FIVE

What Makes Appreciation So Special?

"Some people smile to make friends. Others smile to look younger and live longer. And then there are those who so totally get life, that smiling is all they know."

Alan Cohen

L et's take a closer look at appreciation. Because if it is indeed the key to happy, healthy longevity, we need to know a lot more about how it does that.

1. Appreciation and gratitude

First of all, appreciation differs from gratitude in that appreciation doesn't rely on someone having done something that pleases you, or for something good to turn up in your experience. Gratitude is something you express after the fact—*after* someone gives you a gift, a compliment, a raise, a new car, that whatever-it-is you so wanted. You are dependent on something good happening to you or in your environment for you to feel gratitude.

Appreciation is something you express *before* the fact. Appreciation is a thought, first and foremost, and a thought doesn't rely on anything but your choice to think the thought. That is the critical difference. Absolutely nothing has to happen in your experience for you to think appreciative thoughts. You just have to want to do so, and then focus your attention accordingly.

Your dog can track mud gleefully into the house, and you can think, "Darn! Now I have to mop all over again" or, "There goes my dog! Happy and playful." You have to mop up the mess either way, and you certainly don't have to like the mud, but one choice of thoughts focuses on your annoyance, the other on how much you value your dog's exuberance. Nothing nice had to happen. You didn't have to wait for a squeaky-clean, always obedient pet to turn up in order to appreciate him/her. You simply chose to do so.

Appreciation is about valuing. It is deliberate, conscious attention to that which you value about anyone, anything, or any situation. Including yourself. What's downright miraculous about appreciation, is that *you* are the one reaping the benefits of your appreciation. It isn't the person you are appreciating whose heart experiences a more even, regular rhythm necessarily, it's you! The same result is demonstrated with the brain studies. *You* experience the better functioning of your brain because of your appreciating.

Not only do you not have to wait for anything good to happen so that you have something to respond to, you have direct impact on your well-being just by virtue of your appreciation of whatever it is; yourself, another, a situation. Oh, the object of your appreciation may very well find themselves in a better place because of how you value them, but the first person to benefit is you.

Being valued does, of course, have its own benefits, which is what explains the extraordinary results experienced by the men in the Langer study described in Chapter Two. These men weren't given five-star hotel treatment at the retreat, with concierge service and attendants at every turn. They even had to lug their suitcases to their rooms, something that was a considerable physical challenge for many of them. They weren't given any therapy, physical or psychological. They weren't deferred to because of their real ages, or coddled in any way.

They were, however, appreciated. They were valued as persons able to take care of their everyday needs, and as they discussed various topics, their thoughts and comments were valued. It is that valuing of who they were that accounts for their amazing physical and mental changes.

Appreciation and gratitude enjoy a close symbiotic relationship. It is virtually impossible to appreciate someone or something without feeling grateful for that person or thing. As your dog tracks mud into the kitchen, valuing their "happy, playful" self melts you into gratitude for your dog's existence. How much poorer your life would be without this (albeit messy) being! You certainly can withhold your gratitude on purpose, but if you allow your feelings to proceed naturally, appreciation will inevitably lead to gratefulness.

When you are feeling grateful for something good that happened or that someone did for you, it's almost automatic to appreciate whatever it was, to find value in that something. Which is why, when we say "Thank you" we often follow it up with, "I appreciate it." You are aware, even as you express your thanks, of the value that thing or experience has for you. Even with something as simple as someone saying, "You look nice today," your gratitude for their compliment is followed by a recognition of the value the compliment has for you. It made you feel good, if only for a moment.

So yes, gratitude certainly can lead to appreciation. But since appreciation is a thought you can generate at will, it is the path to gratitude with no "waiting around for good stuff to happen" required.

2. Appreciation attaches meaning

The meaning you attach to an experience defines what that experience will be for you. When a person or experience has positive meaning for you, you appreciate the experience, you value it. And of course, the opposite is equally true.

My stomach doesn't tolerate sharp curves taken at high speeds, a condition I share with one of my dogs, the only difference being I tend to wait until I'm out of the car to let the nausea have its way with me. So if someone proposes a thrilling ride on a roller-coaster, the meaning I attach is one of extreme unpleasantness. Appreciation is the farthest thing from my mind. Someone else—many someone elses actually, given the popularity of high-speed roller coasters—will attach a meaning of extreme fun. They appreciate the experience so much they will wait in endless lines to do it again. And again.

Nowhere was the significance of meaning to appreciation better demonstrated than in the remarkable "Hotel Maids" study.[1] The work performed by the maids in each of two hotels exceeded the thirty minutes of daily exercise recommended by the Surgeon General, a fact none of the maids were aware of. The researchers shared this information with the maids at one of the hotels, including how many calories were burned in the course of each cleaning activity, and not with the maids at the second hotel.

The results? When assessed after one month, it was found that the first group weighed an average of two pounds less, had a smaller percent of body fat, and systolic blood pressure an average of ten points lower, without their having altered their eating habits or exercise routine outside of work (which for most was irregular or non-existent). The second "uninformed" group showed virtually no changes in their weight, body fat or blood pressure.

What happened? The first group of hotel maids assigned meaning to what they were doing on the job, they now appreciated their work differently. These maids were no longer "just cleaning," they were doing something more valuable; they were exercising, with all the positive meaning we attach to that activity. The subconscious message to their bodies, transmitted as described in Chapter Two was, "I'm exercising, get with it!" Their bodies obliged by responding to that mental and emotional message with weight loss, less body fat and lower blood pressure. Yet the maids weren't physically doing anything different.

Such is the power of appreciation. When you value something you attach positive meaning to it, and your mind and body respond accordingly.

3. Appreciation and happiness

Much like gratitude, happiness usually follows an experience, one that generates pleasure. So once again, you're in "waiting for it to happen" mode before you feel happy. However, with happiness, or generating pleasure, we tend to believe we can take charge of the experience: make it happen, so to speak. We go to a movie, or buy an outfit, or eat chocolate, or make love, all of which are great, but the happiness that results is often temporary. You can only go to so many movies in a day, buy so many outfits, gorge yourself on so many chocolates, or find so many willing partners. Not only that, but what gave you happiness one day may not do so the next.

Approached directly in this manner, happiness is an elusive bugger. As long as your happiness depends on something outside of yourself, you're at the mercy of whatever and whoever to come along in order for you to feel happy. However, if you engage in the active practice of appreciation (which we'll discuss in Chapter Six), you will feel the gratitude that accompanies it, and with that, happiness will ensue as night follows day. This happiness you can access any time you wish; it is predictable, reliable, and depends on no one other than yourself to generate it. How to do this is what the rest of this book is about.

4. Appreciation and optimism

Imagine: there you are, appreciating your life, feeling grateful for the experiences and people that make up your world, happy—you can't help but feel hopeful and confident. You are optimistic. Because there's no way you can value yourself, your life and those you share it with, feel that gratitude, allow happiness to unfold—and feel pessimistic. Pessimism, by its very definition, is "a tendency to see the worst aspect of things or believe that the worst will happen."[2]

When you choose to appreciate someone or something, you start from the opposite end of the spectrum. You deliberately look for the positive meaning something has for you, the value it has, which is the best aspect of things, not the worst. It is, in the everyday understanding of optimism, seeing the glass half-full. Appreciation, logically, can only take you down one road: to gratitude, happiness and optimism.

It is indeed the key that unlocks all the other prime components of enjoyable longevity.

Here's how the process goes. Appreciation engages gratitude which together engender happiness, which results in optimism, which leads to greater appreciation, which in turn engages more gratitude which leads to greater happiness and so it goes, an unending cycle of positivity so that yours can be a happy, healthy long life.

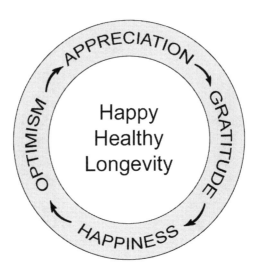

The next step is to take appreciation out of the land of the conceptual and scientific and into the land of the practical and everyday. Because that is what truly matters: how to get appreciation to work for you in your life.

CHAPTER SIX

Hocus Pocus, the Magic of Focus

*"Experience is not what happens to you;
it's what you do with what happens to you."*

Aldous Huxley

Appreciation is, above all, a shift in focus. Instead of focusing on what you don't have, can't do, and aren't, you focus on what you do have, can do, and who you are—right here, right now. You go from "what I don't value" about whatever it is (including yourself), to "what I do value" about the person, thing or situation. It's a deliberate, fundamental, change in perception.

No one illustrates this shift better than the differently-abled. To name but a few: people who, whether from soldiering, birth defects, accidents or disease, are missing one or more of their limbs. The National Wheelchair Basketball Association has both male and female teams that whiz about the court in wheelchairs, valuing their arms, ability to learn and adapt, and upper body strength rather than lamenting their lack of legs.[1] Same with the AMP1, whose motto is "Live fearlessly," the only organized team of amputees playing stand-up (versus wheelchair) basketball in the country, even winning against non-amputee teams.[2]

Then there are individuals such as Dr. Beck Weathers, a pathologist, who at age 50 was caught in a blizzard while climbing Mt. Everest. Despite all odds, he survived, but his right arm was amputated below his elbow, as were all four fingers and the thumb on his left hand, in addition to parts of both feet and his nose. Dr. Weathers shifted his focus and worked with what he had. He figured out how to modify his pathology equipment so he could keep working, and to this day, he practices medicine and travels around the country giving motivational speeches.[3]

Stephen Hawking, the famous theoretical physicist, was first diagnosed with amyotrophic lateral sclerosis (ALS) when he was 21, and he was not expected to live to be 25. Over the years, Hawking has found ways to live and work despite his ever more compromised condition. He has never let it slow him down, even though since 1985 he has had to speak through a computer system, which he operates with his cheek. As of 2015, at 73, Hawking continues to work as director of research at the Cambridge University Department of Applied Mathematics and Theoretical Physics, and has indicated that he has no plans to retire.[4]

What about those who are differently-abled in the mental arena? Peter Leonard, a 54 year old learning disabled handyman, won a seat in the New Hampshire House of Representatives—on his seventh try. The reason? He says, "I wanted to become a pastor. I always wanted to help people. Now I have the whole state to help." Leonard submitted a number of bills to the State Legislature, of which at least one was passed. Leonard didn't dwell on his disability, he forged on, relying instead on the value of his dedication, persistence, and genuine desire to be of public service.[5]

Similarly, the Down syndrome Joey Moss was born with didn't stop him from being inducted into the Alberta (Canada) Sports Hall of Fame in 2015. Moss's story starts when he was working at an Edmonton bottle depot. His dedication to his job inspired hockey great Wayne Gretzky to suggest to the Edmonton Oiler's general manager to give Moss a try. That "try" began in 1985 and continues to this day, with Moss as the invaluable locker room attendant for both the Oilers and the Edmonton Eskimos. Moss's determination and passion for hockey—for which he has received many kudos in his 51 years—have made his Down syndrome irrelevant.[6]

Then there are the long-lived who are shining examples of how much you can accomplish with a simple shift in focus, among them:

Harriet Thompson, age 92, is an exceptional "can do" individual. Thompson made history in June of 2015 by becoming the oldest woman to ever finish a marathon (her 16th); 26 miles in 7 hours 24 minutes 36 seconds. This, despite her being a two time cancer survivor, who wore stockings during the marathon to cover open wounds from recent radiation treatments.

But the most remarkable thing about Thompson is her attitude. In an interview with Mark Strassmann of CBS TV she shared how she thinks about doing marathons: "I'm gonna do it, not I can't do it, I'm gonna do it. And that helps, to be positive."[7] Talk about a shift in focus! Not only does Thompson not dwell on the pain and discomfort of her cancer, she doesn't even dwell on the physical demands of marathon running. She steps into appreciation mode, "I'm gonna do it!" with what she has, her present abilities, and off she goes.

How about Arthur Rubinstein, the great pianist, still playing concerts while in his 90s? When asked how he was managing to do so with such brilliance, Rubinstein replied that he performed fewer pieces, practiced them more often, and—in order to compensate for some loss of speed and manual dexterity—slowed down just a bit before entering a fast passage, which made his playing sound faster than it really was.[8] He didn't bemoan the lack of his previous speed or dexterity, he valued what he had, a vast store of knowledge of how an audience perceives music, to make his playing sound just as accomplished as ever.

Back in the 1990s, a group of gerontologists at Tufts University refused to accept the prevailing notion that once you've hit your late '80s and 90s, it's all over. "People have an unduly negative attitude about what can be done with those at the end of their lives," said Dr. Maria A. Fiatarone, director of several Tufts University studies on the elderly, "We need to be more optimistic."[9] These gerontologists took a group of the frailest residents of a nursing home, of which the youngest was 87 and the oldest 96, and put them on a weight-training program for eight weeks.

The results? The residents' wasted muscles came back by 300%! Their coordination and balance improved, to where some who had been unable to walk without assistance could now get themselves up and to the bathroom unaided in the middle of the night, a source of great personal pride and accomplishment. Not only that, but the "working-out" residents were less depressed, more social, and regained a sense of active life.[10] No mean feat in just eight weeks. All because the researchers' focus was on what the residents could do, not on what they couldn't. The researchers' appreciation of what was possible encouraged the residents to shift their focus to what they could do with the physical abilities still available to them.

There are many other individuals who have empowered themselves by making whatever they could appreciate about themselves or a situation their approach to life, rather than succumb—as many of us do—to what we can't do, aren't, or don't have.

My question to you is: What do you value about aging? About getting older? If you say "Nothing!" you're in trouble. Because that is the crucial question. If what you see before you as you advance through your 70s, 80s, 90s and beyond is deterioration, ill-health and decrepitude, well then, you're in for a very unhappy time, and probably won't live that long. It's scientifically proven.

A study done by Yale researchers asked people then in their 50s or older to agree or disagree with statements such as: Do you think that things will get worse as you get older? Do you think you'll be less useful as time goes on? Do you think you'll be as happy as you were in your youth? Twenty-three years later, it was found that people who viewed aging more positively lived an average of *seven and a half years longer* than those who viewed it more negatively. Simply having a positive attitude made more of a difference on longevity than blood pressure, cholesterol levels, body weight, exercise or smoking.[11]

So yes, we're starting with the question: What do you think is in store for you as you proceed through the years? There's no right or wrong, good or bad answer to this question. There's just your willingness to answer it honestly, for yourself.

It doesn't matter where you are starting from. If right now all you see before you is a depressing sexless future of withered limbs and declining mental status, you can change that perception, you can discover how to appreciate yourself, life and others regardless of your age. With appreciation will come a reason to live long, namely—happiness and enjoyment of life. Because, let's face it, it's hardly worth living long if all you're going to do is be depressed and miserable.

If, on the contrary, you already see a joyous future of fun, adventure, new friendships and love abounding, it can only get that much better as you become an even more expanded, more conscious, appreciator.

Let's take it one step further. What do you think will be of value in your older self? What will you appreciate then that maybe you don't, now?

How about the tremendous freedom to be utterly your unique self? Iris Apfel, for example, at 93, is a fashion world icon. She wears her signature bracelets from wrist to elbow;

her outfits are a riot of bright colors, and her glasses are super-sized with black frames. At 83, Carmen Dell'Orefice, with her high cheekbones and distinctive silver-white hair, is the world's oldest super-model. Yes, you read that correctly. Super-model, not just "model."

At 82, Lynn Dell owns the Manhattan Off Broadway Boutique, which caters to women who refuse to join the invisible brigade of the old and useless. She says, "We are all living longer. We are enjoying our lives. We have a sense that I can do what I want now. I can make a statement now."[12]

What statement would you like to make? John Glenn, the first American to orbit the Earth, at age 41, made his second trip into space at 77 *because of* his age! Glenn observed that many of the changes people go through as they age seem to parallel the experience of astronauts during weightlessness. From that realization, Glenn did his research, convinced others of his idea, and landed a place for himself on the Discovery space shuttle launched in 1998. Glenn used his Discovery journey to conduct scientific experiments on aging.[13] If Glenn had not viewed his age as a positive, something of value, he'd have had no reason to lobby for a place on the shuttle, much less succeed in getting it.

If your perception of your 65-75-85-95-105-year-old-self isn't what you'd like it to be, doesn't have the ring of fun and adventure about it, work on it. Collect examples of people who are enjoying their later years. I have a picture of a very elderly gal doing the splits pinned up on my mirror, which totally inspires me every time I see it. And YouTube is an unending source of older folks doing wonderful things.[14] Once you open your eyes to the fun some 90 year olds are having, you'll be surprised at how much more willing you become to step into that joy yourself.

Critical to shifting your focus in terms of what aging is all about, is the notion of change. From birth—actually from conception—you are changing every second of every day. Imagine if someone told your ten year old self that you would never change. You would be ten forever; mind, body, spirit. For about a minute that might sound good, but then you realize that means you'll be in fifth grade forrrrrever, you'll never be that baseball pro, rock star or fabulous fashion designer you dream of. You'll be ten. Done, finito.

Well, what society calls aging, is nothing more than change. Something you are completely familiar with, given that you've been doing it forrrrrever. When you think in terms of your later years as simply different, changed as was your twenty or thirty or however year old life from your ten year old life, you're able to step away from your preconceptions, and look at "aging" in a whole new light.

At this point, you may be willing to accept that aging isn't synonymous with impending doom, but still believe that you can't become a "glass-half-full" person. You may think of yourself as a realist, meaning you see an awful lot of negativity in yourself, others and the world, and don't really get how you could be any different. Or maybe you believe it's all in your genes. Some people are born happy and some people aren't. Nothing you can do about it.

Not so! For one thing, research shows that all around the world, people are in a mildly good mood most of the time, unless they've just experienced some particularly bad event.

This holds true whether people are rich or poor, in a stable or unstable environment; a mildly good mood is the norm.[15] You're already closer to being an optimist than you may realize.

Genetically, you're less hard-wired than you think. Or more accurately, about 50% (on average) of your being is genetically influenced, and about 50% is a result of environmental factors.[16] Dawson Church, PhD, concludes, "The tools of our consciousness—including our beliefs, prayers, thoughts, intentions and faith—often correlate much more strongly with our health, longevity, and happiness than our genes do."[17]

Can you change your basic personality, say from being introverted to more extroverted, not so nice to nice, lazy to more of a hard-worker? According to recent research, as long as you set concrete goals and make specific plans about how you want to behave differently in certain situations, yes. Such change comes about in increments with diligent practice over time, but yes, change occurs.[18]

Wherever you are on the "positive versus negative person" scale or the "optimist versus pessimist" scorecard, you can become more of an appreciator, one who is grateful and happy, with the subsequent advantages to your longevity.

I am living proof of the possibility of such change. I was eleven years old the first time I attempted to commit suicide. I swallowed an entire big bottle of aspirin (the only pills I could find in the house). My stomach hurt horribly and my ears rang for two weeks, much to the mystification of our family doctor since I certainly wasn't about to cop to what I'd done, but I didn't die. My second attempt was shortly after my seventeenth birthday, when I found out just how difficult it is to smother yourself. I passed out, but that was it. I earned myself several months with a psychiatrist for that one, a first for our family and certainly for me.

At the end of the treatment, the psychiatrist gave me a "to-do" list, and said I'd be all right if I followed his recommendations, but that someday I'd have to deal with the fact that I hated myself. "Doesn't everybody?" I asked. I was perfectly sincere. Anything other than that would have shocked me. My final attempt was when I was in my 20s, and when that didn't work, I figured I was here for the duration, so I might as well try to find a way to get happy. It took a fair amount of therapy, self-help books and a lot of effort, but anyone who has known me over the past 30 years absolutely will not believe that I was ever anything but the happy optimist I am today.

What else? Appreciation isn't something you put off until it hits you, "OMG, I'm getting old!" Appreciation is something to start immediately—whatever your chronological age—and maintain as a habit and practice throughout the rest of your life. As is true of any good habit and practice, the more diligently and whole-heartedly you work appreciation, the more you will enjoy its benefits in terms of your longevity and health.

Finally, appreciation must be sincere. Your brain responds to the electrical energy of thought, not to actual words, so whatever is the thought behind your words is what will trigger the transmission of chemicals throughout your body. If you state your appreciation of the wonderfully health-conscious meal your mate prepared for you, but you're thinking, "This better be good for my health because it tastes dreadful," your brain responds to "tastes dreadful," not to your kind words to your significant other.

The same holds true of gratitude. If you thank your brother-in-law for the holiday sweater he gave you, no matter how profuse your thanks, if what you're thinking is, "This has to be the most garish thing I've ever seen, and he's beaming! He's so pleased with himself, I could just puke," your brain will ignore your thanks and internalize your criticism. The one person you can never lie to is yourself, so don't bother.

The next section is composed of tools and techniques to help you develop the practice of appreciation in your life. Some are told as stories, others as straight-forward information. This is not an attempt to show you all the ways in which you can appreciate—that's impossible—but rather to give you a sufficient variety of specific real life examples, making it easy for you to apply one or more to yourself or to your life circumstances. The goal is to make appreciation an effortless go-to regardless of what is happening in your life, regardless of the situation, so that you can enjoy the happy, healthy long life you deserve.

With that, game on!

PART II

What You Need to Do

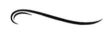

1.

∞∞∞

Step Away From the Comparison Game: Be Grateful to Be You!

HARRIED, BEDRAGGLED, ALREADY late for work, you do your best to be patient as your three grandkids scramble out of the car juggling school backpacks and soccer gear, when the youngest pipes up, "Where's my lunch?" Oh, shoot. In the fridge, that's where his lunch is. Why on earth you volunteered to take care of the kids while your son and daughter-in-law went on a two week vacation, you have no idea. Oh, now you know why. You'd forgotten how much work kids are.

You root in your purse, grab some bills and shove them at your grandchild, "Sorry, Sweetie. Here's some lunch money. Gotta go. I love you." As you maneuver your way out of the cramped school drop-off area, you glance over to a sleek SUV, driven by an equally sleek woman.

You grind your teeth. How does she do it? She just dropped off her three charges, just like you, but unlike you, she's unflustered, her car is immaculate, she's immaculate—hair, makeup, everything perfect and in place. You could kill her. Or yourself.

You go to work. Your manager walks into your workspace, collects your latest effort, sweeps a critical eye over your habitual mess and says, "It'd be nice if you got your projects in some semblance of order." "I get the work done!" you announce defensively. "Yes, I know. Think of how much better you'd do if you could find things more easily, like Lynn," your manager says, smiling to ever-neat Lynn as she leaves. Lynn smiles at you. Pertly. You'd love to stick your tongue out at her, but she'd probably just smile at that too. Retirement can't come too soon.

You feel less than, defeated, diminished. Your sense of self is pathetic. Your appreciation for who you are, for what you do accomplish in your life? Oh, please. You'd like to stick your tongue out at me too!

Before you succumb to a full-on pity party, how about an appreciation check? The reality is that you are a fine human being, with your own set of talents and skills. You accomplish what matters to you, as best you can, from where you are at the time. The reality is that the only thing defeating you is your comparison of yourself to others. And frankly, comparing ourselves to others is damning every time.

It doesn't matter whether you come out smelling sweet or smelling icky, comparison can only hurt. Your current "I'm not good enough" choice (as a grandparent or a worker) causes stress to invade your mind, heart and body, leading eventually to diminished health and well-being. The opposite, "They're not good enough," may feel good in the moment, but over time only leads to pain, personally and in your relationships—another source of stress.

Step away from comparing yourself to others. Period. If someone exhibits a behavior you admire, work on adopting it for yourself, but don't judge yourself for not already having that behavior.

Focus on those of your talents, skills and behaviors that you are proud of. Appreciate how very valuable they are to you, how meaningful they are to your home life, your work, your relationships. Tend to your mental, emotional and physical well-being by being grateful for your skills and talents! Buff them up, shine them to a high gloss, use them well.

Be grateful you are you! It's a much surer road to happiness, and wonderful for your happy, healthy longevity.

2.

——————— ∞∞∞ ———————

The Lion King and Aladdin Get the Best of a LaGuardia Situation

TRAVEL DELAYS ARE never fun, but from time to time they are bound to happen. You can't expect the weather to cooperate every time you fly, and better they should repair those mechanical issues before you fasten your seat belt.

I've learned to take a deep breath, chill, remind myself it's not the end of the world, and then look for a way to appreciate whatever extra time I'm now spending in the airport. Reading always works for me, so does getting in some phone-chat time with girlfriends, or cleaning out my inbox if all else fails.

But recently, the Broadway cast members of *The Lion King* and *Aladdin* took appreciating your unanticipated downtime in an airport to a whole new level. During their six-hour weather delay in New York's LaGuardia Airport, they had a sing-off! It was truly an extraordinary event, captured on someone's phone, and uploaded to YouTube [https://youtu. be/6ajHZWDP_Vk].

What a choice these cast members made! Rather than bemoan the hot, crowded conditions of the airport, rather than complain endlessly about what the delay meant to their plans, or how bored they were, or anything else, they turned to what they could value in that moment, they started singing. First one, then another, then the whole cast of *The Lion King* joined in to sing songs from their award-winning show. Whereupon the *Aladdin* cast responded with their songs—including an amazing free-style rap by James Inglehart, who plays the Genie in the show.

Not only did the cast members of these shows counter the potentially adverse effects of negativity on their well-being, they uplifted everyone within earshot in that airport! You can see the smiles on other passengers' faces as their mood changed from "Oy ve" to "Hurrah"! Because everyone was in the same weather-delay boat; it took deliberate, conscious focus to switch from ain't-it-awful to better thoughts and feelings. Something the cast members accomplished with ease.

Contrast this with the behavior I witnessed a few weeks prior at another airport. My flight was mechanical-issue delayed for three hours, then canceled entirely. We were transferred to a different flight, which meant another delay of about two hours. OK, such is life. Finally, we were in line to board our designated aircraft, just waiting for the previous passengers to get off the plane and the few minutes required for the cleaning crew to do their thing.

60 | Noelle C. Nelson

A man standing at the head of our line was vigorously complaining to the ground attendant in charge of taking our boarding passes about how long it was taking the previous passengers to deplane. How he'd had it with all this waiting, and what a horrible airline this was, and what horrible service. There was more of course. I stood there, with my jaw dropped. Here the airline had kept us safe (off a plane not fit to fly), found us seats on another flight, we were about to board, and the man was first in line. It was probably one of the finest examples of complete lack of appreciation I have ever seen. At the very least, the man could have valued his position at the front of the line, and appreciated the fact that he only had another ten minutes, tops, to wait before getting to his seat.

I don't even want to know what that man's heart condition is like. What I do know, is that those Broadway cast members, with their ability to switch their focus to what they could appreciate, what they could do—sing!—as opposed to what they couldn't do (get on a plane right then) had their hearts not only in the right place for the joy they brought themselves and everyone else in that airport, but also in the very best place for their long-term health and vitality.

Now don't you wish you'd had *that* travel-delay?!

3.

Shape Your Life Up: Tell Yourself the (Desired) Truth

ACK!! YOUR COMPUTER is acting up—again—and despite hitting "escape" and every other "get-me-outta-here" key you can think of, you're in frozen hell. "I hate this computer!" you sputter. Your significant other glances over at you, "That's what you always say. Maybe you should try talking pretty to it." You snort, "Right! And the computer can hear me and will suddenly unlock itself." Your mate shrugs, "Works for me."

You grumble and groan, finally give up and power down your computer, knowing you'll lose that last bit you so meticulously labored over. You figure you'll run some errands and have another whack at the computer later. You stop off at the market. "Not that I'll be able to find a good parking spot," you mumble, "Not in this rain." Five complete rounds of the parking lot later, you jam your car into a too-small space all the way at the far end, under a tree you're certain will drop sticky goo all over the car, and trudge into the market. Wet. You left your umbrella at home. "Figures," you snarl.

Sure enough, there are a couple of sticky goo blobs on the windshield. You wrestle your dripping bags into the car and bang your knee as you sidle into your seat. By the time you get back home, you're not fit company for anyone. Not even your cat, much less your family.

What happened here? Is your life destined to be no more than a series of irritating events? Well, maybe yes and maybe no. It all depends on what you're willing to tell yourself about whatever is going on. Because whatever you tell yourself is what will shape your perception, and perception is what determines action.

Before you say, "I have no idea what you're talking about" and hit delete, read on just a little further. It will all become clear.

Minds are funny things. They respond to suggestion, which is actually direction. When you say, "I hate my computer!" your mind looks for things to hate about your computer. When you say, "I won't be able to find a good parking spot," your mind rushes to obey. It does that by focusing your attention on those things that will fulfill your own prophecy.

With your computer, it doesn't occur to you to phone your friend Mike, generally thought of as computer-savvy, for his help because your attention is locked (just like your computer) on "hit a key and get out of this." At the parking lot, your attention is fixated on "won't find a parking place" so you don't see the customer slip into her car, ready to exit. You forgot your umbrella because you repeatedly say to yourself, "I always forget my umbrella," which your mind promptly acknowledges by focusing your attention on locating your keys and away from the umbrella stand as you head out the door.

What about your health and longevity? How do you talk about that? You come across a group of kids having a blast rollerblading, doing twirls and jumps, laughing the whole time and you say, "Oh, I could never do that. I'm too old." Your mind hops to it, "Got it!" and focuses your attention on your creaky knees. You watch a couple dance a sinuous tango and sigh, "Ah, the good old days." Your mind bows to your wish, and reminds you of everything else you used to love and never do anymore.

Your mind is, at all times, a willing servant. All you need to do is give it different direction.

Say to yourself, "Things always work out well for me" and deliberately focus your attention on what is working out well for you, or what could. Your mind will get the hint after a while, and start looking for things to work out well for you. You revel in the roller-blading kids' delight and think, "That looks like fun." Your mind focuses your attention accordingly, "There's that roller-skating rink over by the market. Roller-skating's easier than roller-blading, safer too. Think I'll give it a try." You admire the tango dancers, "What grace! What flexibility!" Your mind focuses your attention in that direction, "Mary is taking a stretch class. I'll bet if I joined her, I could get back into some kind of dance."

Over time, you will see more and more ways in which things are working out well for you (or could), and they will work out well for you much more of the time. You've changed what you are able to perceive in what's around you.

The key to working with your mind is to talk to yourself genuinely, believing that what you are telling yourself will soon be true, just like when you said, "I hate my computer" or "I could never do that. I'm too old," you said it with absolute conviction.

Train yourself to talk differently, positively, to yourself. You'll be amazed at just how quickly your mind responds, and how your experience of your life shifts into a much happier place, the precursor to enjoyable long-life.

4.

Turn "Yeah, but" on Its Head

EVER HAVE ONE of those "Yeah, but" conversations? Your friend has lost her job. At 55. Being the supportive friend that you are, you say:

"Hey, you've got tons of skills. All you need to do is revamp your resume, and you'll be hired in no time."

"Yeah, but the job market's over-crowded with Millennials and kids fresh out of college. How am I gonna compete against that?"

"Piece of cake! You've got tons of experience, and you've got personality and smarts on top of skills."

"Yeah, but what if that's not enough? You hear stories all the time about people like me who can't catch a break. Apparently we're too old and "over-qualified"!"

"Those are just urban legends. People like you, with all

you've got going for you, you'll find an even better job in no time."

"Yeah, but what if I don't? How am I gonna pay the rent?!"

"Well, I'll help. And so will the rest of your friends, you'll be OK. It's just a transition time."

"Yeah, but…"

It's a conversation with no end. Your friend has now driven herself even deeper into her depression/fear/anxiety hole, and you're increasingly frustrated, since all your good will and good ideas are met with "Yeah, but."

You may or may not eventually get through your friend's "Yeah, buts" but one thing is for sure; you can get through your own "Yeah, buts" with a slight change in focus.

Oh, you thought this was going to be about your friend? Sorry. That was just an easier way to ease you into remembering all the times you've allowed the "Yeah, buts" to destroy your confidence, dreams, hopes and desires, and along with that, loaded unnecessary harmful stress on your present and future well-being.

Because that is precisely what negative "Yeah, buts" do.

You have a dream of having your own business. Something you can start now and rely on for as long as you want to keep working. Maybe on the Internet. Your internal dialogue goes something like this:

"I'd love to create a fantastic app/clothing/game—my own business."

"Yeah, but, who are you to do something like that? People

way smarter and younger than you are failing at that one every day."

"I know, but maybe I could. I mean, Steve Jobs started in a garage."

(Peals of laughter from the committee in your head.)

"Yeah, uh-huh, you are soooo like Steve Jobs."

Turn the tables on the negative "Yeah, buts"!

"I'd love to create a fantastic app/clothing/game—my own business."

"Yeah, but, who are you to do something like that? People way smarter and younger than you are failing at that one every day."

"Yeah, lots of people fail, but lots of people succeed too— at any age! I could be one of those."

"Yeah, but—you hardly have the smarts to do that."

"Yeah, maybe there are other people who are smarter, but smarts and youth aren't everything. I've got perseverance and passion in spades! I really want this and that counts for at least as much as smarts."

Get the drift? Instead of killing your hopes and dreams with negative "Yeah, buts" emphasizing all that you can't do, nurture and support your dreams with positive "Yeah, buts" strutting all that you can do.

Your immune system will thank you, your brain will function oh so very much better and your heart will sing your praises. How's that for a giant step towards both your success *and* your happy, healthy longevity!

5.

Getting Your Nursing-Home-Phobic Spouse to Help with Mom

YOU FINALLY HAD to move your mom from her home into a skilled nursing facility. She never recovered properly from the fall she took last winter, and despite her fierce desire to remain independent, it became obvious even to her that calling you in the middle of the night to help her get off the bathroom floor wasn't a good long term plan.

Your husband helped with the move: pitched in to box things up, do the garage-sale number on what was left, even helped fix up your mom's house to facilitate the sale. You thanked him profusely, you were beyond grateful.

But when it was time for that first visit to the nursing home? Screech! Halt! Suddenly your "I'll always be there for you, babe" guy wasn't there. At all. He dug his heels into the ground, "I don't do nursing homes." Oh, great, so now what? You have to do it all alone? "She's your mom, babe. I did what I could. I'm done."

And with that, your anger grows. You start noticing all the other things that dear old hubby does that annoy you. Piss you off. Are downright obnoxious. That you've put up with for all these years because he's your husband. And you love him. Hmm. Not so sure about that right now!

You're full bore into resentment and a cold sullen mood that never seems to lift. It's all his fault. He's uncaring, non-supportive, non-compassionate and every other non-whatever you can think of.

But with all that, he's fine. Meaning he's going about his life just fine. Your mom is in the nursing home, adjusting to it pretty OK. The only one who is unhappy is—you! The resentment and criticalness that have taken over your being are even now damaging your health, and with it, your prospects for healthy, long life.

Should you paint a "Little Mary Sunshine" smile on your face and pretend all is hunky-dory? No. But you might try having a real conversation with your husband instead of a blame fest. You might try asking him what he would be willing to do to help you out.

For example, you tell hubby-dearest what your responsibilities are. You shop for the toilet paper, tissue, shampoo and whatever else your mom wants. She doesn't like what the nursing home provides—no big surprise there, she's always been fussy. You talk with her on the phone three or four times a week. You pay whatever additional costs the nursing home/

insurance doesn't cover. Once a week you drive the hour it takes to get to the nursing home, more if the traffic kicks in. You visit with your mom for about an hour. You drive back.

Having laid it all out, you ask your spouse, "What would you be willing to help me with?"

Much to your surprise, he doesn't just blow you off. Hubby sits there, thinking. Then announces he's willing to do the shopping if you're too busy or too tired one week and provide him with a list. He'll pitch in some bucks to help with the uncovered costs. He'll even make the drive with you. The one thing he won't do is actually walk in the nursing home and visit with mom: "Hospitals and nursing homes, babe. Can't do 'em."

You have a choice now. You can graciously accept and appreciate the help offered, or you can beat him up (mentally/verbally!) for not actually visiting with your mom. Graciously accepting relaxes your mind and body, allows your immune system to function better, and puts you back on track for a happy, healthy long life. Beating him up, even if only in the deepest recesses of your mind, disrupts the smooth functioning of your heart and brain to your detriment.

Graciously accepting and appreciating means you can look at the situation more constructively. What's to say you can't do something fun with hubby-dear after the mom visit, rather than just turn around and drive straight back home? He can do something he enjoys during that hour visit; catch up on a ball game, or whatever else. Rather than resent the situation or each other, you both can seek to make the best of it—and of each other.

Your life. Your choice. Make it a happy, healthy one!

6.

Smile! It's Good for Your Health

IT'S BEEN A bad-dream of a day. You overslept, you had to hurry through the dog's early-morning walk—during which he refused to poop, but then promptly pooped as soon as you got back in the house—your hair-dryer died in a brief evil-smelling flash, you forgot to get gas and had to wait in a ridiculously long line at the pump. Your boss has a new favorite (it's definitely not you), the team meeting dragged on interminably, and you only got half your work done.

You came home to a messy house that still smelled vaguely of dog poop. You burnt dinner, your spouse was cranky and bedtime couldn't come soon enough.

Sound familiar? Well, here's an easy quick way to find relief. Smile! No kidding, smile. Recent research shows that "smiling can reduce the level of stress-enhancing hormones like cortisol and adrenaline while increasing mood-enhancing hormones like endorphins" (Ron Gutman. *Smile: the Astonishing Powers of a Simple Act*). Science-dude words for "smiling makes you feel good" in real we-can-measure-it bodily terms.

Children smile about 400 times a day. Some 67 percent of adults smile less than 20 times a day, and on a day like the one you had? Chances are you barely cracked a grin even once.

Unfortunately, just slapping a smile on your face without a feeling of enjoyment or appreciation behind it won't work. Plus, you'll feel really silly flashing a fake grin that shows teeth and little else. But you can find genuine reasons to smile throughout your day: quick easy scientifically proven ways to lower your stress literally dozens if not hundreds of times a day.

How? By being deliberate. By proactively looking for something that gives you pleasure or that you can appreciate, right here, right now.

For example, you overslept, the dog pooped in the house, your hairdryer died, and all the rest, but you're finally on your way to work. Now find whatever reason you can to smile. Listen to an amusing or uplifting podcast. Appreciate that you have a job. Appreciate that you have a way to get to work, appreciate that you are finally on your way. Admire the plants that miraculously manage to grow right at the edge of the freeway. Notice the sunny day, or appreciate how warm and dry you are as the clouds presage rain. Dwell on whatever gives you even a moment of pleasure and allow that pleasure to spread through your being into a smile, a wonderful boon to your health and well-being.

All through your day, deliberately seek out the people,

situations, thoughts and memories you truly appreciate, that lighten your spirit, that make you smile. Today, and year after year, smile your way into happy longevity.

If all else fails, watch a cat video. I kid you not. Researchers at Indiana University have found that watching cat videos boosts your energy, promotes positive emotions, and decreases negative feelings [http://bit.ly/1JXf09h]. I defy you to watch kittens being adorable (or puppies, or baby goats, or hedge-hogs, whatever your preference) without cracking at least a hint of a smile.

You will find greater ease, you will find relief, your body, mind and spirit will all benefit from the simple expedient of looking for—a smile!

7.

What Improv Theatre Taught Me About "Yes, and"

YOU'RE PLANNING YOUR next vacation. Well, your only vacation this year, which is a pretty big deal because you and your significant other haven't had one in, oh, let's see—quite a while. It should be a delightful discussion, after all, you're talking about something you both want and are up for.

The conversation goes roughly like this:

"Let's go to the beach."

"We always go to the beach. I want to go hiking in the mountains."

"What do you mean, we always go to the beach? And anyway, you had a hiking trip already."

"Well that was just for a weekend—this is different!"

Instead of a pleasant discussion, you end up feeling defensive, put upon, dissed. You know what's coming… a fight.

Why? You're both grown-ups here. What happened?

You felt attacked. Your "hiking" idea was shot down. You retaliated, whereupon your partner got defensive and so on. All very understandable knee-jerk reactions, however, nothing that will lead to what you really want: a solution. More than that, a mutually agreeable solution.

When I started classes in improv acting, I was surprised to discover the first rule of improv theatre is "Yes, and." No matter how outlandish the situation your fellow improv actor presents on stage, your response has to be "Yes, and." "Yes, puppies do grow on Mars and we should think about starting a Martian kennel. I'll get right on building that spaceship." Refusing a partner's offer is known as "blocking." A blocking response would be: "That's ridiculous, anyone knows there's no life on Mars, certainly nothing like puppies." The scene stops right there, because it has nowhere to go.

Your partner says, "beach." You block with, "We always go to the beach." And the conversation promptly goes downhill. Instead, practice "Yes, and." "Yes, we do go to the beach often, and I think a change of pace would be fun. How about maybe trying out some mountains-and-hiking this time?"

Your partner may come back with, "Well I don't know. The beach is really my preference." You continue with, "Yes, beaches are great. What if we found a lake with a beach area and a hiking area?" Or whatever other creative solution you come up with.

In other words, you're now into problem-solving, being

creative together to find something that pleases both of you. You can't do that when you're busy protecting your own territory.

"Yes, and!" Whether you actually use those words, or just the spirit of them, is a great way to both honor yourself *and* your partner's preferences. It's yet another tool in your arsenal of easy-to-use, always available appreciative techniques, the building blocks of your happy, healthy longevity.

8.

━━━━━━━━━⚬⚬⚬━━━━━━━━━

Become an Optimist in Three Easy Steps

YOU'RE CONVINCED. BEING an optimist is the way to go. But beyond the old adage "See the glass half full" how do you do it?

Here are three quick, easy steps to becoming an optimist:

1. Play the "What If" Game Positively

We all play the "What if" game, but for the most part, we play it negatively. For example, you haven't been feeling at all well lately. It's not a cold, not indigestion, nothing you can put your finger on. Your mind starts spinning, "What if it's cancer? I'm getting older, maybe it's diabetes? Or something leading to a stroke? Heart attack?!" which leads to, "What if it's already too late? What if I've got something terminal? What if they can't figure out what it is? What if I don't have enough insurance?"

Panic sets in, and with that, your stress increases as your ability to think clearly and make good decisions goes directly downhill.

Instead, play the "What if" game in a hopeful, positive, appreciative direction: "I've been in pretty good health all my life. It's not like I'm in pain even, I just don't feel as well as I'm used to. I've always bounced back from things, I've got good stamina. This is probably a vitamin deficiency, like vitamin D or something like that."

2. Appreciate What Is

Appreciate what is. You have good access to doctors and other health-care providers. You have endless access to Web research. You can remind yourself that our 21st century ability to treat most ailments is sensational, that all sorts of diagnostic tools and techniques exist to ferret out what's going on with our bodies. At least you have insurance! And you have friends and family who could help out if the need arose.

All this reassures you that the sky isn't falling right this second, which helps you relax, assuring that you are functioning at your least-stressed best. You can now be proactive and approach your health concerns in a more rational, logical way.

3. Reminisce Constructively

Most of us, when faced with a situation we don't like, reminisce destructively. We think of all the bad things that have happened to us, how awful it felt and how hard it was to get back on track.

Instead, reminisce constructively. Deliberately think about how easily you healed from that broken leg you got falling out of your treehouse at age 12. How whenever you get a cold or the flu, it never lasts more than a week. How you can't even remember when you last had a headache. How good you feel most of the time.

Think of all the good health advice friends, doctors and untold others through blogs and webcasts have given you along the way. How you always seem to have been shown the way to happy, healthy well-being throughout your life.

Now, if in addition to these three steps, you should feel the urge to not just become, but to flourish as an optimist, to embrace optimism mind, body, heart and soul, then do your best to live the Optimist Creed (http://www.optimist.org/e/creed.cfm). It is a powerful appreciation practice that can literally transform you, inside and out, making your happy, healthy longevity practically inevitable.

The Optimist Creed

Promise yourself:

- To be so strong that nothing can disturb your peace of mind.

- To talk health, happiness and prosperity to every person you meet.

8.

- To make all your friends feel that there is something in them.

- To look at the sunny side of everything and make your optimism come true.

- To think only of the best, to work only for the best, and to expect only the best.

- To be just as enthusiastic about the success of others as you are about your own.

- To forget the mistakes of the past and press on to the greater achievements of the future.

- To wear a cheerful countenance at all times, and give every living creature you meet a smile.

- To give so much time to the improvement of yourself that you have no time to criticize others.

- To be too large for worry, too noble for anger, too strong for fear, and too happy to permit the presence of trouble.

9.

Terrified of Getting Older

WHAT IS IT about getting older that terrifies you? Why does turning 40 or 50 or 70 (!!) makes you depressed and anxious?

I'm standing in front of a restroom mirror, fixing my hair, and a 40-something woman is groaning as she looks at her reflection. "I hate this," she says, speaking to no one in particular as she touches up her makeup, "No matter what I do, I can't look any younger." She crumples up the tissue she was using to blot her lipstick and turns to me as she tosses it in the wastebasket, saying, "I don't know why God invented getting older. It's like some sort of cosmic bad joke, you know?" As she walks out of the restroom, I think, "Well, it depends on your point of view."

The more you think getting older means getting useless, or worthless, and therefore unwanted—by the opposite sex, by employers, anyone—the more depressed and anxious you will be, which will have a decided negative impact on your happy, healthy longevity. Instead, approach each milestone, whether that's 40 or 60 or whatever, recognizing your increased value at this new point in time.

Lots of qualities only appear as you get older: wisdom, patience, a sense of perspective and understanding. Many other qualities like caring, a sense of humor, self-confidence also frequently increase with age. And no matter how old you are, find people older than you are who can inspire you. Believe me, there are plenty of those around once you start looking! Then, you can actually look forward to each coming year.

Age is only frightening if you let it be. True beauty, grace and courage just get better over the years.

10.

I Should Have Married A Mind Reader!

YOU AWAKEN TO the decidedly irritating noise of a vacuum cleaner or the lawn mower, take your pick. You squint at the clock. It's 6:30 a.m. on a Saturday morning. Groan, moan, pillow over head. You try to get back to sleep but you can't. You sit up, feeling annoyed, resentful and guilty all at the same time. Lovely. This is gonna be one of those Saturdays. You flop back down on the bed trying to figure out escape maneuvers into some peace and quiet.

In any of this, do you communicate effectively with your significant other, source of the above irritations? Highly unlikely.

If you're a guy, you probably yell, "Can't I get some peace and quiet around here?! Is that too much to ask?" If you're a gal, you probably dish out a healthy dose of the silent treatment for the next few hours, punctuated with martyred looks and sighs.

All because you don't want to ask for what you want. Oh, you're willing to demand or manipulate, but how about just plain old ask?

"My mate should know what I want by now! We're not new to this relationship, it's been 5-10-20 years. Can't my supposed sweetheart have the slightest bit of consideration for what I need, for what I deserve, without my having to ask for it?"

Maybe. In fairy tales. But as you no doubt figured out early on, real relationships take more than the wave of a wand or some magical thinking. They take communication of all sorts, including speaking up for what you want. Appreciate it! Value the fact that you can open your mouth and have a reasonable discussion with your mate about things. Recognize that all your Saturday morning happiness depends on, for example, is a switch in focus from your present "woe is me" stance to an empowered and empowering "let's talk about it."

Having to ask doesn't mean your mate doesn't love you, it simply means he or she is not a mind-reader. Which is a good thing, because let's face it, you probably wouldn't want them actually reading every thought that crosses your mind. Requiring them to be a mind-reader is crazy-making. Even if your beloved can pretty much guess what you want, chances that they'll get it right every time, or time it just right aren't good. They'll feel like a failure, and you'll still be unhappy. Not a good scenario.

Switch your focus. Quit your martyr/victim routine, step

up to the plate and take responsibility for what you want, need and deserve. Engage your mate in a friendly, loving dialogue where you assume that he or she really wants to be there for you in every way, and that you can—together—always work out ways to satisfy most of what you both want and need.

"Honey, I'll be happy to help you with the chores on Saturday. Do you think we could maybe not get started until around 8:00? I could sure use the extra rest. I'll bet you could too."

No, you won't get what you want all of the time, but you'll get a lot more of it more often. Most importantly, you won't be grinching and irritated, with the subsequent ill effects on your long-term health and well-being, because you'll know if something isn't working for you, you can talk about it, you can ask for how you'd like it be different.

What a relief.

11.

Put Grit in Your Personal Goals

PERSONAL GOALS MAY be easy to set, but hard to achieve—as anyone who's resolved to get in shape, stop smoking, or vowed to get to work early every day can attest to.

The first few days are a breeze. Off you jog to the gym, so proud of yourself. You toss your smokes in the trash, yippee! You get to work, a little bleary-eyed, but early enough to get a good head start on your day. All is well.

Fast forward to a month later. You're still on track, sort of. You don't exactly jog to the gym, but you get there. Most of the time. You've bummed a cigarette off a friend a couple of times, but that's all. You're getting in early to work once or twice a week. Not too shabby.

But by four or five months down the road, forget about

it! You're depressed and down on yourself. Are you doomed to the big "L"?

Hardly. You just lacked "grit." "Grit" is research psychologist Angela Duckworth's word for what separates those who succeed magnificently in life from those who just do OK. Grit is passion plus perseverance. According to her research, many talented people do not succeed because, despite their talent, they lack grit. They may have passion, but no perseverance. It seems the ability to just keep going (cue Energizer Bunny) really does make the difference.

I remember when I first started dancing, gazing in awe at the accomplished dancers twirling around the floor. I asked my teacher: What makes them so amazing? Is it raw talent? Body shape? Particular training or technique?

She told me that all of these things mattered, but what made the difference between a good dancer and a great dancer, was that the great dancer practiced, practiced and practiced some more, regardless of the day of the week, the dancer's mood that day, or whatever else might be going on in their lives. They had passion—the love of dance—and perseverance.

So, if you really want to see your cherished goals, your ardent aspirations, through to success, first of all, choose something you are passionate about. Something you can fall in love with. If it's a healthy body, great, if it's clean lungs, great, if it's improving your sales performance, great. It doesn't matter what the goal is, what matters is that you absolutely unequivocally, adore it. That you value and appreciate what it will do for you, that you are enraptured by how meaningful it will be in your life.

Your steadfast focus on the tremendous benefits of your goals to your life will not only make perseverance much easier, it will assure that you receive both the future well-being you desire and well-being all along the way. Instead of a stressful journey, you embark on a hopeful, happy one, which can thus contribute to your happy, healthy longevity.

Secondly, in the abiding words of the classic Nike ad: "Just do it." Day in, day out. No excuses. Persevere. Use whatever you need to motivate yourself. I personally love cheesy success posters and recite endless affirmations. Find whatever inspires you and use it.

Grit works. Work it!

12.

────────── ∞∞ ──────────

My Way or the Highway. Really?!

YOU'RE DOING THE dishes. You don't mind doing the dishes. It's kind of a relaxing thing for you. You drift and think about your day as you scrub; about how you're going to resolve that situation at work, you remember a funny thing you heard on a podcast earlier. "Why are you doing it that way?" your partner asks, interrupting your reverie. "Huh?" you respond. "Why are you scrubbing the pot that way?" your significant other repeats, more insistent.

"I don't know," you say, staring down at the pot, "I've always scrubbed it this way." "Well, that's dumb. You should do it this way," your partner replies, and in no time at all, you are in the middle of a "my way is better" argument in which each of you is trying to convince the other of the best way to scrub a pot.

Or, your friend is planning a fundraiser for the local animal shelter. You think how inefficient their approach is, and you tell them, "You shouldn't do it that way, do it this way." Once again, in no time at all, you find yourself in yet another "my way is better than your way" argument which leaves both of you unhappy and feeling out of sorts. Your friendship suddenly doesn't feel so friendly.

What's going on here? What's the problem? Well, let's face it, each and every one of us thinks our way is better. As a matter of fact, each and every one of us thinks it should be obvious to everybody else that our way is better. Now that wouldn't cause problems if we would keep our opinion of "better" to ourselves. But we don't. More often than not, especially with loved ones, friends and co-workers, we take up the cause of "my way is better" and try to force our righteousness onto our fellow man. Appreciation, valuing that which matters to others, isn't even in the ballpark.

If someone asks you for your help or advice, or if you are in a teaching position relative to them (instructor, supervisor, boss), or if you are functioning in a professional capacity where your advice is sought (i.e., accountant, manager, dentist, doctor, counselor), that's fine, it's totally appropriate. But when you're just going about your life, dishing out "my way is better" to those around you whether they asked you or not, you're setting yourself up for some very poor relationships.

Happy, healthy relationships provide you with a low-stress environment, very conducive to happy, healthy longevity. One of the keys to such relationships is acceptance and appreciation of the differences between us. One of the hardest things for humans to do is accept and appreciate differences. No wonder so many of us find relationships difficult! Yet relationships free of "my way is better" are possible, if you will keep the following guidelines in mind.

- Different is just that, different. Different is not better or worse. Different is just different.

- People do things in different ways, go about things differently, approach life differently, because these ways work for them. These may not be the most efficient, or smart, or elegant ways to go about life from your perspective, just as how you go about life may not be the most efficient, or smart, or elegant way from someone else's perspective.

- Observe. Pay attention to how your friend, spouse, partner goes about their life. Ask questions. Learn how and why this particular approach or way of doing things works for them. Seek to understand rather than to criticize.

- If you want to do something together that the two of you do differently, figure out how your way can fit *with* their way, not how your way can replace their way. Tell them what you are doing. Enlist their help! "I want to watch TV with you. I enjoy being with you, and chatting about the shows. You love to channel surf. I'm more comfortable watching one show. How can we work this out together? What are your ideas?"

- Listen to what your friend/partner tells you. Look more for what will work than for what won't.

That is appreciation at its finest. It's valuing that which has meaning, that which matters, to someone else as well as to yourself. Be willing to change your ways, not to sacrifice how you do things, but to explore new possibilities. Be willing to appreciate the many ways of going about the "doing" of life, and recognize that yours is only one of them.

13.

⊶⊷

Taking Those Car Keys Away: With or Without Drama?

I'LL NEVER FORGET the day I knew I had to take the car keys away from my mom, then in her 80s. I was waiting outside for her to come back from the market. She turned in from the street, missed the driveway completely, and drove right onto the front lawn. She stopped the car, got out, looked down at the grass under her feet, then up at me and said, "Your father's going to kill me." I didn't know whether to laugh or cry. My dad had been dead for almost a year.

Yet, even with that unprecedented event, mom stubbornly resisted my attempts to get her to stop driving. She insisted it was a "once in a lifetime" occurrence, and indeed, although mom had always been what my sister and I called a "jerk and stop" driver, with a heavy foot on both gas and brake, she'd never had an accident. And she knew her husband was gone, it was just the shock of what she'd done that momentarily discombobulated her. Still, she had to give up the car keys. But before she would acquiesce, we both had a lot to learn.

1. The Value of Independence

Having a car, whether it's a second-third-hand beat up old clunker, or a zippy smart car straight off the production line, is an enduring symbol of American independence. It's what lets you go where you want when you want however you want, and most of us will do practically anything to get that first set of wheels. No big surprise it's a life-changer when we have to give them up!

I couldn't take away my mom's independence, it meant too much to her. So I looked for other ways to preserve it. I discovered the many resources like "Dial-a-ride" and minibus door-to-door transport services. I found out that AAA has a foundation for traffic safety which offers advice for caregivers, and that AARP has guides for every state on transportation alternatives. I came to appreciate what was available to help mom call the shots on her comings and goings, rather than having to call me every time she wanted to go somewhere.

2. Provide Training Wheels

I don't know about you, but I thought training wheels were the best invention ever. OK, so I was six, but the transition between tricycle and bicycle was terrifying. Training wheels made all the difference.

Helping mom appreciate a different approach to getting herself to wherever she wanted or needed to go was just as terrifying. Intellectually she had no problem with the idea of calling up a service to book transportation. She wasn't in love with the idea, it wasn't as easy as driving herself, but she accepted it. Emotionally, she was as panicked as six-year-old me.

So I became her training wheels: I went with her the first few times. Once she saw that she really would get where she wanted to go, and that there were people to help her get on and off the minibus if she needed it, that the vehicles were clean (what can I tell you, she had her standards!), and that the drivers were nice—she managed just fine.

Yes, I occasionally did "dutiful driving daughter" gigs when mom had an appointment that made her particularly anxious, like certain doctor visits, but overall, mom was coping well. Would she rather have still been driving? She groused about it from time to time, but she also said it was a relief not to have to worry about driving onto the lawn.

We both came to appreciate what was possible, what was workable, instead of dwelling on what wasn't, much to the betterment of both our states of health and happiness.

My mom still had most all her wits about her when she passed, quietly and without fuss, a week before her ninety-fifth birthday.

14.

Want Success? Focus on What Works

YOU'RE ANNOYED WITH yourself. Very. Downright angry, now that you think about it. You vowed last month you'd stick to your newly created budget, and save up so you could get the plumbing fixed. Yet here you are, berating yourself over the shoes you had to get, on sale—no returns.

Which wouldn't be so bad except for the expensive lunch you treated your niece to at the latest "in" eatery because you forgot her birthday and felt guilty about it. And there's the hair loss treatment "as seen on TV" you splurged on, which so far hasn't nurtured a single follicle.

Deep mournful sigh.

You're a failure. A spineless, totally lacking in self-discipline failure. At least that's what you tell yourself. Can't stick to a budget, not even for a measly four weeks, even with the potential reward of a toilet that flushes reliably and doesn't embarrass the heck out of you when friends come over. Might as well give up. Who'd want you as a friend anyway?

Oh, for heaven's sake. Put your violin down and appreciate what really happened. In your month, you succeeded at following your budget twenty-seven days! That's fantastic! Why would you give your three "off" days more credit than your twenty-seven "on" days?

Yet that's exactly what we do—with our money management, quality time with our kids, work projects, our love lives—we give inflated, exaggerated, overdone credit to our goofs, our flubs and our mistakes. We pretty much ignore, dismiss, or otherwise devalue our successes.

What a recipe for disaster! Whatever you focus on grows. If you choose to focus on your mistakes, your supposed "failures," you dump into a poor-me focus, which only increases the likelihood of your making more and more of these flubs, as well as stressing you out. Given that hopelessness, depression and aggravated stress wreak havoc with your well-being, you've just skewered your chances for happy, healthy longevity for no good reason.

Instead, accept that "OK, that wasn't the swiftest choice for me to make" when you mess up, and simply come up with a new plan that makes it easier for you to be successful. Keep your focus steadily on the many times you did reach your stated goal, appreciate them, and get on with it. You get on with it by moving on, not by standing in place and stamping your feet all over your suffering self-esteem.

Focus on and value what's going right with your budget,

in your love life, your work life, whatever it is you want to improve, and not only are more successes bound to come your way, but you'll increase the happiness and well-being in your life with no added effort.

15.

Tip Your Marital Scales Into Joy

YOUR HUSBAND WAKES up grumpy, stumbles to the bathroom, glances at your reflection next to his in the mirror and says, "What's wrong with your hair?" You glare, "I slept on it funny. Good morning to you too."

"Why does he have to be so unpleasant first thing?" you mutter to yourself. Strike one against husband.

You're trying to convince your squirming cat that getting her flea medication applied really isn't the soul-crushing, humiliating experience she makes it out to be. Your spouse enters, clean-shaven, ready to go. He holds out his car-coffee-cup: "We're out of coffee." "So, make some," you reply, chasing cat #2, who's not having any, seeing what cat #1 had to endure.

15.

"What am I, your slave?" you think. Strike two against husband.

Mid-day, with too much to do and too little time, you text your mate, "Pic up dry cl plz." He texts back, "OK." He breezes in at 6:00, gives you a squeeze and a kiss, plops down on the couch. No sign of any dry cleaning. You ask, "Did you leave the dry cleaning in the car?" "Oh, forgot to pick it up. Sorry, babe." Cheers sports on TV.

"You thoughtless, selfish pig!" You barely manage to strangle the words so they won't come out of your mouth. Strike three against husband.

By bedtime the mood is decidedly chilly. He's definitely out. No cuddles from you tonight, that's for sure.

Could this unfortunate end to your day have been prevented? Other than by trading your husband in for the mythical Stepford Husband?

Yes, indeed it could, simply by following the famous 5:1 rule. Namely, for every one negative thought or statement about your spouse, you need to balance things out with five (yes that's right, FIVE) positive thoughts or statements. No, I didn't pull that figure out of thin air; it's been well established, first by Dr. John Gottsman's research (*Why Marriages Succeed or Fail*), then by many others.

Here's how the 5:1 rule plays out in real life:

Pulling from our example above, when you have that "Why do you have to be so unpleasant first thing?" thought, you'd do your best to find five things you appreciate about your spouse to counter it. It could be—that it's nice to have

110 | Noelle C. Nelson

a spouse! That at least he notices your hair. That he's usually pleasant in the mornings. That maybe he had a bad night, he'll get over it. That your hair really does look funky, he's right, and you can have a laugh over it.

See how easy that was? And I don't even know your husband.

When you pile negative thought on negative thought throughout your day—or your marriage—you destroy the good that is there. Choose instead to deliberately look for positive, appreciative thoughts about your husband or your relationship.

Constantly tip the scales in favor of what you appreciate rather than what you don't, and you'll reap the delicious short and long-term benefits of happiness and joy.

16.

Waste Not, Want Not

YOU LOOK AHEAD to the rest of the year, and you're scared. There, you've said it. It's out in the open, you're scared. Your situation has never looked this bleak. Sure, you still have your job, but given the recent round of layoffs—most of whom were Boomers, just like you—for how long? Raises and promotions are out of the question (forget about a bonus) and you weren't at the top of the "boss's fav" list to start with.

You groan, drop your head in your hands. No more spontaneous nights out with, well, anyone. No more keeping up with fashion or gadgets this year. No more lattes (OK, maybe one a week). You reach slowly for junk mail you fished out of your mailbox when you got home. Coupons. You'll clip more coupons, watch for sales. "Waste not, want not," your mother always said. You vow not to waste a penny from this day on. Not a penny, not a dime, certainly not a dollar.

But what about life? What about a vow not to waste a

single moment of that precious gift we call life? For when we treat ourselves or others with anything less than respect and compassion, we are trashing life. When we spend our time (the currency of our lives) blaming others, refusing responsibility, holding grudges, we are wasting our life. When we forget to look around us with appreciation and profound gratitude for all the good (persons and things) that make up our life, we are wasting our life. Waste not, want not, is a profound *life* truth, not just a financial caution.

Don't wait for New Year's! Right here, right now, make a vow, a resolution worth the commitment with the determination to see it through. Vow that from here on in you will look for the good, the positive in yourself and in others and dwell on that. Vow that you will look for the opportunities in every situation and every encounter. Vow that you will see silver linings everywhere and dismiss the clouds.

Vow to embrace life with appreciation and joy at every turn, and your life will be filled with yet more to enjoy and appreciate. Waste not a precious moment of your life in negativity and you will never want for happiness in all the coming years of what's now bound to be a healthy, long life.

You smile. Waste not, want not. Maybe clipping coupons isn't such a drag. Maybe it's just another opportunity in disguise.

17.

Be Truly Human: Practice Random Acts of Kindness

REMEMBER THE SLOGAN "Practice random acts of kindness"? It's been around for a long time, all the way back to the early '80s. More often than not, it was dismissed by most folks as a cute New Age aphorism and has largely been forgotten in the years since. Certainly in our hurried, harried hyper-technological age, we hardly have enough time to accomplish our daily list, much less engage in random acts of kindness.

Yet, random acts of kindness are what nurture the humanity in us, prevent us from turning into mindless texters and tweeters, and remind us of the true nature of humankind: that we are all in this together.

Take, for example, a story that generated major social media buzz. Suzanne Fortier, a Panera Bread store manager, made clam chowder for a call-in customer's cancer-ridden grandmother on a day when the chowder isn't usually available, and included with it a gift of cookies from the staff.

That was a classic "random act of kindness." There was nothing in it for Fortier. If anything, she had to go to the effort of making chowder and someone ended up paying for the cookies somewhere along the line. Yes, the story went viral and no doubt Panera Bread will acquire some new customers because of it. But that isn't why Fortier made the soup, nor is it what's important here.

What Fortier did, was to be kind to someone who needed a little TLC. A stranger, yes, but a fellow human, and it's reaching out to a fellow human in a caring way that says "we're all in this together." It's yet another way to value and appreciate those with whom we share our lives, be that for just a moment, or an entire lifetime.

Random acts of kindness are easier to practice than you may think. You can practice a whole host of them without it costing you a dime or any real effort.

For example, smile at people when they pass you on the street. Say "Have a nice day" as you exit the elevator. Allow someone who's in an obvious hurry, or trying to deal with a cranky child, to cut in before you at the supermarket checkout. Refrain from yelling at the customer service person on the phone. Let them know: "It's not you, I'm frustrated with the situation." Comment (appropriately please!) on someone's cute hat or nice shoes or well-polished car when you're filling up at the gas station. Tell the barista how much you appreciate the care they took with your coffee.

These random acts of kindness and many more like them

are easy to do. And they restore a sense of caring and connection to each other as we go about our busy lives. All such acts will cost you is a moment of attention to the other human beings inhabiting the same planet as you do, trying as valiantly as you are to make it through another day.

Add a moment of unexpected kindness to their day and you will experience a moment of unexpected joy in yours. Moments of joy added to moments of joy equal more moments of joy, all contributing to your increased health and well-being until there you are, living the happy longevity you always wanted.

18.

∽⊶∾

A Non-Waste of Time Team-Building Exercise Worth Trying at Home

YOU MOAN, YOU groan. The fired-up 30-something go-getter manager the higher-ups unleashed on your department has called one of his infamous "team-building" meetings, and it's only the threat of getting fired that propels your butt out of your chair and into the meeting. What a waste! Sitting around doing departmental Kumbaya when you have piles of work marked "Urgent!" and "Rush!" on your desk.

It isn't exactly in a mood of eager anticipation that you park your unhappy self in the meeting room. Mobile devices are strictly forbidden, so you don't even have the distraction of mindless browsing, tweeting or texting. You wish you'd learned the art of napping with your eyes open, especially when your manager announces his latest and greatest team-building exercise.

He states that he wants the team to work more closely together, to think of each other more as family than as co-workers. And you're thinking, "Right. As in highly dysfunctional family." He goes on to say that each team member has a particular strength they lend to the team, and that if each team member would bear in mind and appreciate their teammates' strengths, the team would function better as a whole. A highly cohesive unit. He states he will now point out what he feels is each team member's strength.

Oh great, you think, he's gonna tell us who the movers and shakers are and pin a woeful L on the others. Like we didn't know already who his favorites are. You stifle a yawn and pray for this to be over soon.

Your manager turns to the guy you consider by far the most innovative and creative in the bunch, and says, "Your strength is energy. You bring tremendous energy to whatever project you're engaged in." You're surprised. You would have thought he'd laud this guy's innovations.

Your manager turns to another team member and says, "Your strength is your "whatever" attitude." You smirk inside. Yup, he's gonna nail the L on this guy, who was born with the sarcasm gene. But your manager takes a different route. He says, "You don't jump up and down enthusiastically, but you never complain. You say "whatever" to the task you've been assigned and take it on."

You sit up and take notice. Your manager's right. That is how Mr. Whatever behaves. Your manager defines another's strength as "playfulness" and appreciates how that individual lets in new ideas. You listen differently now, as your manager appreciates, not work accomplishments or the lack thereof, but something positive, something of value about the essence of every person on the team. And he's right on, every time.

Your manager concludes by stating that he wants each team member to think of the others in the light of these strengths, to focus on what each member can appreciate about the others. Darned if that isn't exactly what happens! You start looking at your co-workers differently, not in terms of what they can or can't do for you, how successful they are at this or that project, but rather what value their "energy," or "whatever" or "playfulness" brings to the mix and how that does make the whole team function better.

In addition, you discover, much to your surprise, that you're happier at work, as you dwell increasingly on what you value and appreciate about each of your co-workers—and your manager! Your well-being improves as a result.

You decide to use your team manager's approach with your family, your friends, your significant other: heck, even with yourself. You have fun playing the "What's great about you?" game with all those in your life, instead of the tried-and-tired "What's wrong with you?" game. There's an unexpected bounce to your step and more often than not, a smile on your face.

Then it hits you. You're doubling up on your chances of happy, healthy longevity by appreciating both at work and at home. Smart cookie, you!

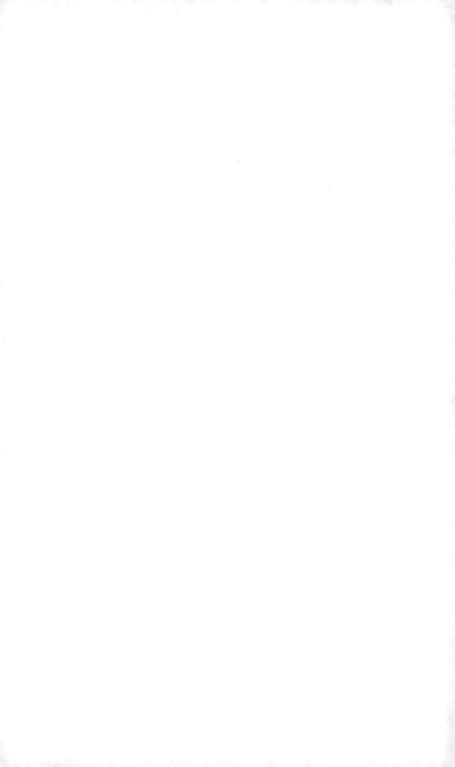

19.

Living in "Can't Do/Don't Have" Mode? Try Living in "Can Do" Mode

YOU'RE ANNOYED. YOU promised yourself you would lose that weight and go to the gym so you could join your friends in a much vaunted walk-a-thon. Yet here you are, six months later, one month away from the walk-a-thon, and you've only lost a couple of pounds and gained nothing in terms of muscle or stamina. You're starting to make up excuses to give to your friends.

But what could you do? Work takes up most of your time and energy, and family eats up what's left. Who has time to work out when there's dinners to make, chores and errands to do, grandkids to sit, elderly parents to tend to and all the rest?! Not your fault, you try! And who can resist a little comfort food now and then to soothe the day's irritations? OK, a lot of comfort food, but what's a body to do?

You're mad at yourself for ever agreeing to join the walk-a-thon, and yes, it's for a good cause, so of course you feel guilty about shining it on. Plus your friends are counting on your participation and you hate disappointing them.

Let's review. You feel pissed, depressed, guilty, and you're still not up for the walk-a-thon.

Or are you? Right now, you're clinging so tenaciously to the problem—what you can't do, don't have and aren't up to—that you have no hope whatsoever of resolving it.

Rather than complaining, fault-finding and blaming, none of which get you any closer to either the walk or feeling good, try thinking appreciatively about the situation and working toward a solution.

Step 1: Accept What Is

You're not going to get in shape or lose all the weight in one month. It's OK. It doesn't make you a bad person.

Step 2: Focus on What You Can Do, Be, or Have Right Now

You can lay off the comfort food and increase your intake of fresh fruits and vegetables or whatever else enhances your overall health. No, not to lose the weight, but to feel better about yourself.

You can get to the gym once a week, or do some low-key stretches and exercises at home several times a week, or go for a walk around the neighborhood for a half hour every other day or evening (take the dog, he'll thank you). Not to whip yourself into shape, but again, to feel better about yourself.

Step 3: Go for a Doable Solution, Rather Than an In-Your-Dreams Solution

Accept the likelihood that you won't be able to walk side-by-side with your friends and go for something you *can* do, rather than just giving up altogether.

For example, engage your sense of humor. Tell your friends how great you think they are, how much you appreciate their inspiring vim and vigor, and that you'll be gawking at their fine form from behind. Way behind.

Or, join your walk-a-thon group in support. Volunteer to man one of the water tables, or help set up, or stand at a critical place along the walk and cheer them on. Be at the finish line to welcome your friends with water and huzzahs!

Living in the problem—what you can't do, don't have and aren't—gets you nowhere. Living in the solution—what you can do, have and are—may not get you your ideal outcome, but it will get you a potentially very satisfying and self-esteeming one that is far better for your long-term health and joyous well-being.

20.

What I Learned From Yucky Fish

WE'RE GREAT AT giving our very best in the hard moments, the crises. We pull out all the stops to save a loved one's life, rescue a child from a burning building, salvage our marriages on the brink of divorce. We are truly, then, the shining example of what a human being is capable of.

But what about in the more mundane moments? The day to day. How often are we giving our very best at those times?

I was at dinner with my sister and brother-in-law recently: their treat. The conversation was pleasant, the restaurant very nice, yet most of my focus was on the dry, unappetizing fish entree I was politely eating.

It wasn't until later that evening, as I was driving home, that I realized I hadn't given my best to the evening. I hadn't even given a quarter of my best to the evening! Instead, I'd given far too much of my attention to the three square inches of poorly prepared, overcooked halibut on my plate.

What a waste! I'm not saying I should have fallen in love with yucky fish. I am saying that there was so much more to that evening, and had I been giving my very best, I would have shined on my dislike of the fish dish (it's not like I'm starving, nor that it was my last meal), chalked it up to "not gonna order that again," and turned my focus and attention to all that was there to enjoy and appreciate; my sister and brother-in-law, the pleasure of being together, the nice restaurant atmosphere.

When we give of our very best, we appreciate. We love. We care. We value what matters, versus indulging the piddling little complaints that eke away our joy and threaten our chances of happy, healthy longevity.

Don't wait for life-threatening events to hit before you rise to your very best. Give of your very best, as often as you can, throughout your day. Notice and be grateful for what there is to appreciate at work, with your family, your friends, your hobbies, with yourself.

The more we give of our very best, moment to moment, the richer, happier and better our lives become. And then yucky fish hardly matters at all.

21.

Want More Life Satisfaction? Supercharge Your Work

YOU'VE GOT YOUR work down to a system. You've been doing it so long that you know what to do, how to do it, and get your assigned tasks and duties done well (for the most part) and on time (for the most part), regardless of whether you're assigning your "to-dos" to yourself or you have a boss who does that. You get that cost-of-living increase most years, or your customer base grows a little every year, so all should be well.

Yet you're plagued by an undercurrent of dissatisfaction. It all seems so hum-drum. Like you're on a pleasant but oh-so-predictable treadmill. It's not bad, but it's not the stuff dreams are made of. But you don't want to work fifty times harder than you already do, thank you very much. You don't want to sacrifice every waking moment of your life to "the job" (much less go out and find a new job) and you need the income, so quitting isn't an option. You groan, hunker down, check what's next on your list and ignore the gnawing sensation of boredom and futility in your stomach.

What if I told you that the solution is available right here, right now? That there is a way to supercharge your work and re-discover a powerful feeling of purpose and worthwhileness, without taking a single seminar, reading (yet another) motivational book, or buying someone's miracle product.

All it takes is asking yourself the simple question: "What is my value to my work, right now?" You see, your value to your work changes over time. When you first start, your value to your work is to show up and to learn how to do certain tasks. Later, your value to your work is to do those tasks with proficiency, and perhaps show others how to do them, or assist others in doing their tasks. What's your value now? How can you contribute, given your level of experience and expertise, in ways that others might not think of?

For example, if you're an employee, perhaps your value would be that you can see ways to do things more efficiently or productively than they are now being done. You can demonstrate that value by offering suggestions, recommendations, even coming up with presentations designed to show the worth of your ideas. Many ideas that power corporations and companies to new levels of success have come from those in the trenches. But first you have to believe in your value and be willing to express it.

If you're your own boss, in the beginning years all you

cared about was having enough clients/customers to put food on your table. Later, your value was in improving your offering. Maybe your current value is in having a sufficient loyal client or customer base that you can approach them to find out, "How can I better serve you?" so that the ideas for how to quantum leap your business come from end-users' experience of your product or service.

Don't let yourself be a work-hamster! Get off the treadmill of "always done it this way, always been this way," and explore the wonderful unknown of "What if?" The more you invest of your own value into your work, the more value your work will have for you. Instead of contributing to your angst, unhappiness and early demise, your work can become a source of happiness and life-satisfaction (key to longevity!) that powers your well-being in the many years ahead.

22.

―――――――― ⚬⚬⚬ ――――――――

Why Me? Every Woman's Lament

YOU GLARE AT the Toad-on-The-Couch your man has become. For years, you've been subtle—"suggested" and hinted and sighed loudly—only to progress to complaining, nagging, fuming and yelling when subtlety doesn't shove him off the couch and into doing what needs doing. Not that your complaining-nagging-fuming-yelling works all that well either.

What, oh what, ever happened to the guy who used to pitch in willingly with whatever tasks were at hand, that prince of a guy who couldn't wait to get home to you, who'd have meaningful conversations with you, and was eager to participate in every aspect of your life?

He's been toaded. Yuck. You want your prince back! Yet no matter which relationship book you pick up, no matter which blog or podcast you turn to, the advice is always the same. You're the one who has to do the work of revitalizing the relationship.

You're sick of it. "Why is it always the woman who has to make nice, make the changes, do the work?" you exclaim, "Why can't *he* get his butt in gear and do it?"

Because *you're* the one who wants the change. He's not the one who's irritated and complaining. He's perfectly content with things as they are. So yes, you're the one who gets to do what it takes for change to occur. Notice I say "gets to" not "has to." Because doing what it takes is an honor, a privilege! It is an opportunity to exercise your personal power. That is a blessed and wonderful thing.

I know you don't like this approach. I know you resent "having to be the one to do all the work." But you see, trying to make him change hasn't been successful. For all the criticizing, nagging, prodding and anger you've displayed, your Toad has sat square on his couch, more resentful than cooperative. Sure, once in a while he budges to do what you ask: mostly to get you to quit nagging. But there's no sustained effort because who likes to be nagged into anything?

Now if your guy were the one wanting the change, I'd be saying to *him*, "You want it, go get it!" I'd be telling him not to wait on you to magically transform yourself, but for *him* to do what it takes. So this isn't a male-female thing. It's a whoever-wants-things-to-be-different-gets-to-take-the-initiative thing.

Science is now proving in a variety of realms what philosophers and spiritual leaders have long known: like energy attracts like. In other words, when you expect the best, and act according to that expectation, you're more likely to get it.

Optimistic happy people tend to attract better health, longer life, and more enjoyable life experiences. Companies with "Best Places to Work" status have employees who are more productive, motivated and present. Couples who appreciate each other rather than criticize, who seek to understand rather than blame, have happier relationships.

You have the power! When you shift your focus to appreciating your man rather than picking at his flaws, express your gratitude rather than taking him for granted, and seek to understand his different ways rather than attacking him for them, good things happen. Think of it as priming the pump, which, as long as there is still love between you, encourages him to become, once again, that prince he was during your first years together. He retreats less and less to his Toad-on-The-Couch behavior. He responds to your change.

When you feel you shouldn't be the one to make the change, you abdicate your power. You place yourself in the weak and vulnerable position of having to wait for someone else to make a change before you can enjoy the benefits of the change you seek. Which means you may be in for a veeeery long wait. Whereas, when you are proactive, when you have the courage to step up and do what it takes to make change happen—why then, change does happen and *you* are the one who reaps the benefits.

So quit complaining about being the one who has to make the change and recognize how powerful you are when you take the initiative to appreciate, be grateful, and communicate rather than criticize! You get results, both in terms of a better, happier relationship and the increased well-being and longer life that goes along with good relationships. That's success. That feels good.

Go for it! You'll be all smiles.

23.

Is It Your Mood or Your Attitude?

MAYBE IT'S THE tooth that's been bothering you that had you tossing and turning, or your mate's incessant snoring, or the neighbors' all-night partying. Who knows? Whatever it was kept you owl-eyed staring at the ceiling, until you finally took a sleeping pill and woke up groggy and cranky this morning.

Then of course you had to rush to get out of the house on time—which you didn't, so you hit more traffic than usual—which made you late. Your boss, who generally doesn't amble in until 10:00, made it in early and wants to know why the heck you're late, and is this how you usually behave? Maybe he pays you too much...

The lousy mood that was creeping up on you since your dismal wake-up this morning is now full-blown. If you could, you'd turn right around, go home, and bury your head under the covers. And it looks like the day is only going to get worse.

You are irritated, angry, crying "unfair" and "why me?" at the universe. You snap at your co-workers, at yourself. You have no patience and seem to be all thumbs. You can't wait for this grinchy day to end so you can go home and bury your head under the covers. Which you probably can't, because when you get home there will be more demands of one kind or another on you. Grumble, grumble.

It doesn't have to be this way. Really! Your mood is generally brought on by physical conditions. You're tired, hungry, cold, or in some other type of discomfort. How you *respond* to your mood, however, is a matter of attitude.

You can choose your attitude, and your attitude is what determines how others respond to you. If your attitude is one of "I feel awful, the whole day is shot," or "I hate feeling like this, I hate being late, I hate being off my game," then indeed, you'll be struggling mightily through your day. Not only that, but a sucky attitude means that your brain, heart and overall body systems aren't functioning as well as they could, precisely when you need to be, if not at your best, at least at your "better."

If, however, you let yourself off the hook with, "I feel pretty awful now, but once I've taken my shower, I'll feel better. Maybe I'll treat myself to a special coffee, that'll up my mood," and similar thoughts, you'll start to feel better. You may still be tired, but you won't plummet into "lousy mood." If you hit traffic, you can simply relax and tell yourself, "Traffic happens, somehow we all get where we need to be going. I'll be OK," and listen to that amazing audio-book you never seem to find time for.

When you walk in to work and your boss has her hissy, you'll be in a much better place to say, "I'm sorry. I'm usually on time. I'll stay later tonight if you want me to" without falling into that "Ain't it awful, woe is me" place. Your switch in focus will not only increase your ability to navigate the rest of your day with more ease and efficiency, it will also give your body and mind the advantage of greater well-being, and with that—a far more certain path to happy, healthy longevity.

The better you can take care of your physical self, the more likely your mood will be good. When your physical being isn't up to par, for whatever reason, boost your mood. Make deliberate choices about your attitude, look for things to value and appreciate, and focus on those as much as you can.

Your day (and your life!) will go surprisingly well.

24.

How to Make Worry Your Friend (!)

THE IDEA OF worry as being anything even remotely "friendly" may seem absurd, yet every emotion has both a positive and negative function. Every emotion has value in your life, something about it that deserves your appreciation. Sadness, for example, as beautifully portrayed in the box office hit *Inside Out*, has both negative and decidedly positive consequences for Riley and her family. Unfortunately, when it comes to worry, we usually see only the negative side, which is to make us increasingly anxious about everything.

For example: "The traffic is awful, what if I don't get there in time, I'll bet my outfit is going to be a wrinkled mess from sitting so long, they're going to think I'm totally unprofessional." "What if I'm too old to find love again, I'll be lonely and miserable forever." "What if I go to that party and I don't know anyone there and I'll feel stupid and I won't know what to say," and on and on. We worry about everything from the vitally important to the clearly absurd.

The problem is, we're not using worry to its best advantage. Worry does have a positive function, a beautiful and wonderful function. It is a warning signal, an internal feedback mechanism that tells us, "Hey, pay attention, there may be some danger here." Used properly, worry is very valuable.

So, how do you use worry properly? With appreciation: heed the warning! Let worry be your friend, alerting you to potential problems, and figure out possible solutions before you go into the situation.

Before you go off to that important meeting, think: Is the traffic likely to be bad? Should you consider an alternate, perhaps longer, but less hassled route? If you are likely to be in the car a long time, choose clothes that won't wrinkle, or remember to hang your jacket in the back. If despite all your good efforts, you are late, have you thought of the best, most professional way to present your lateness?

If you are worried you'll end up alone and unhappy, learn about how to create a satisfying relationship from where you are now. Look for role models of others your age who *have* found love again. Put yourself out there, take the necessary steps. If you are worried about not knowing anyone at a social event, figure out topics of conversation that are of common interest, and decide that this is a great opportunity to make new friends.

Worried about something for which you can't figure out solutions on your own? Ask for help. Ask as many people as you need to, then sort through their different ideas and choose the one that feels best to you.

Once you have figured out practical, workable solutions to your worries, drop them. Just let them go. If the same worries drift through your mind, remind yourself, "I already dealt with that." If they keep drifting through, then use an imaginary fist of white light to POW! those worries right out of your mind.

Hanging on to worries you've thought through is the mental equivalent of letting the alarm clock ring once you're up: annoying and useless. Plus there's the slow but inevitable toll it takes on your healthy well-being, eroding away that happy longevity you so want to enjoy.

Worry is a great friend when you need it, but a big drag when you're just carting it along for the ride.

25.

$$\equiv \!\!\!\!=\!\!\!\!\infty\!\!\!\!=\!\!\!\!\equiv$$

Let Go or Get Dragged

YOU COPE PRETTY darn well with the crises and emergencies of life. Somehow you get through them, over them, and get on with life.

But then there are things that aren't crises, yet somehow manage to irritate, annoy or aggravate you every time you bump into them. Things you don't get over because they're in your face time and time again.

You know, like that ex with whom you had the misfortune to birth a perfectly wonderful daughter who now has kids of her own that you have to "share" with him. And yeah, OK, it's been 20-odd years since the divorce and you've gone on with your life, but every time you see him, you bristle. Your recurring refrain is, "What a jerk!"

Then there's your sister or co-worker or workout-buddy who has this irritating habit of interrupting you before you've completed your thought. Or—better yet—has this infuriating need to tell you what you "should" do at every turn. As if you were a two year old who couldn't put her shoes on the correct foot!

As understandable and as justifiable as your reactions are, they are hurting you more than benefiting you.

Oh, sure, it feels good to roll your eyes at your ex's bad jokes and worse comb-over, or text your girlfriend the gory details of how your sister insulted you yet again. But at the same time, you're stressing your heart, your immune system, and you're probably feeling pain in your gut as well.

That's what negative emotion does to us. Study after study shows that anger, aggravation, and constant annoyance do bad things to your body and your mind.

So what's the answer? To stuff your negative emotions, "Hi! I'm fine!" when you want to strangle someone? Certainly not.

The answer is: feel and release. Feel your hurt/angry/resentful feelings powerfully for five-ten-twenty minutes tops! Confide them to a journal, scream them into your pillow, yell them full volume in your car with the windows rolled up, but then *let go*. Be done with them.

As recovery groups have said succinctly for many years: "Let go or get dragged!" Because that's exactly what your negative emotions will do to you if you hang on to them. They will drag you into unhealthy places. They will disrupt the smooth regular beat of your heart, the full functioning of your immune system, your digestive system, the very way your brain functions.

Once you've done your releasing, whenever you encounter the irritating person again, let their irritation roll right off you. Say to yourself, "Oh, it's no big deal. That's just the way they are." Don't take their comments personally, even if the comment is personal. Let it go! They want to be critical mean people? Not your problem. You can just smile and ignore the barb.

Yes, you can. You are strong enough for that. Remind yourself of the good things you're doing for your well-being, and let go! You, and your long term well-being, are much too valuable to get dragged.

26.

Attitude of Gratitude? (Yeah, Right...)

YOU'VE BEEN IN a frightful mood these past few weeks. The assisted-living housing you found for your dad is eating far too much of your paycheck, not to mention your savings. You're just covering expenses and practicing the fine art of "Which credit card do I max out now and who do I pay before my credit is totally ruined?" A game you thought you'd left behind in your 30s.

Not only that, but you've heard rumors tweeted and face-booked that your company is considering more layoffs. Surely the next to go will be the older employees (read 50+) who cost more in salaries, health insurance and benefits. If that happens, you're looking at the very real possibility of having to sell the home you've loved for so long and downsize to something more affordable. As in tacky and cheap. Great.

So when your co-worker Miss Perky bounces in, gleaming from her pre-work jog, and flashes her immaculately whitened smile at you, saying, "Tut-tut, I see a gloomy face. Where's your attitude of gratitude?" you feel a roar of displeasure coming on.

OK, so you don't roar. It's actually a whimper as you stare resolutely down at your desk, clutching the work you can't seem to get started, and think nasty thoughts like, "Attitude of gratitude, my *%^*! Like I have anything to be grateful for…"

Well, you do, although it certainly may not seem that way right now, and the more you focus on what you can appreciate, what has meaning and value for you right now, the more grateful you will feel, and the more quickly and easily you will lift yourself out of your current woes.

You see, when you are consumed with thoughts of doom, you don't see the opportunities for success and joy all around you. Appreciation and gratitude are not merely cute buzzwords. They are very real perceptual choices, which in turn open up very real options for you. You can choose what you pay attention to in your environment. What you choose to pay attention to has consequences.

When you expend all your energy worrying about your diminishing funds, you're not looking for ways to improve the situation. Like renting out a room in your home, or turning your craft hobby into a source of extra dollars. You're not considering that you might like a smaller place that requires less upkeep. That not all smaller, less costly homes are tacky.

Your worry becomes a self-fulfilling prophecy. When you are riveted by tales of imminent company disaster, you are not doing all that you can to make your job—and yourself—so valuable to the company that you'd be the one person retained despite massive layoffs. If anything, by trailing your misery behind you moaning, "It ain't fair" and "Why me?" you make yourself that much less attractive an employee.

Appreciating what you have, the good or positive that is already in your life, is a way of seeing the opportunities that abound to help you achieve whatever it is you want. Your attention shifts to what is possible, what might be helpful or useful to you in your present circumstances.

So yes, especially when the situation looks foreboding, when it seems circumstances are against you, rouse yourself to an active search for "What could I appreciate here? What could have value for me? What possibility can I be genuinely thankful for?" and go for it with all the energy that the anticipation of success and joy can bring.

Attitude of gratitude? Yes! The sweet path to a healthy, long life.

27.

Are You Listening Competitively? Or Listening to Learn?

YOU KNOW HOW you can be going along in a conversation with a friend or a loved one and it all seems to be good? But then suddenly, you say something and the conversation stalls or stops entirely. You're thinking, "What happened?" You didn't say anything insulting or mean, you just voiced your opinion. Or so you think...

I had lunch the other day with a dear friend I hadn't seen in a long time. I was bemoaning the tediousness of air travel—TSA, the delays, crowded conditions and all the rest—and I said how I would love someday to turn left instead of right when I boarded the plane. Namely, to saunter into the first class cabin where surely conditions were far better than in economy, my usual haunt.

My friend, who traveled extensively for work before her retirement, said, "You know what I used to do? I'd buy my coach ticket, but then, at the last minute, right before boarding started, I'd go up to the counter agent and ask if there were any first class seats still available. And often, they'd say 'yes!' and I'd only pay an extra $200 instead of $2000 and get to fly first."

I immediately retorted with, "Oh, that would never happen now. They jam the planes so full, there's never an available seat to be had."

And with that, the conversation ended: at least that part of it.

It was only later that it hit me. I had unwittingly denied my friend's experience of life. I had flat out slammed my reality in her face, as if her's didn't matter.

There are few things worse that we do to our friends and loved ones than make them feel like they don't matter, that we don't value their point of view, appreciate the way they've chosen to live their lives. We rarely mean to, yet we do it all the time. It would have been so easy for me to consider her experience in my response: "I never thought of that. I wonder if it would still work, given the general overcrowding." I would not have thus denied either her experience or mine. And there would have been a continuing basis for conversation, had we wished to do so.

Simply put, instead of listening *competitively*, "My experience is more right than yours," "I know better than you do about this," we need to (I need to!) listen to *learn*. Listen to those we care about with an ear to: "What does this mean to them? How did they experience it? What about it did they value? How did they come to appreciate it? What about their experience might broaden my perspective?"

Relationships are about caring and sharing. What better way to do both than to appreciate those we love by listening to learn, which benefits not only your relationships but also your long term well-being!

28.

Collateral Benefits: Be Good to Your Mate, It's Good for Your Health

YOU'RE IN THE middle of a screaming yelling fight with your mate. You can feel your heart racing, your blood pressure rising. After the fight, even though you smoothed things out, your stomach is still a mess. You think, "I can't do this anymore. This is just not good for me!"

Or it's that daily litany of things that irritate you about your relationship: the annoyances you put up with, the little things that grate on your nerves, like his snoring, or her never quite putting away all her stuff. His overly loud laugh when someone says something he thinks he should laugh at even though he doesn't think it's funny, or her forgetting to mail the bills on time. You never quite feel relaxed, you tense up every time he/she does it again, your digestive system suffers and you think, "I can't do this anymore. This is just not good for me!"

You're absolutely right. It isn't good for you. When you feel angry, or even chronically irritated or annoyed, you put unnecessary stress on your heart. Parts of your brain shut down, and your immune response weakens. All in all, not a pretty picture.

"Well, now what?" you ask, "Leave my mate to preserve my health?" No, of course not, unless your spouse is abusive, which is a whole different subject. But what you can do, is focus your attention more on what you do like about your spouse, what you can appreciate about what he or she brings to the relationship, to the betterment of your life, and less—much less—on what you don't like, on what has little value for you, and frankly annoys you.

For example, appreciate that he voices his opinion. Turn your attention to trying to understand why he has an opinion so radically different from yours, rather than angrily defending your position. Appreciate the inevitable good that will come out of working things through rather than screaming them through.

Appreciate the emotional warmth and comfort of sleeping by his side. Look into solutions for his snoring. Take a step back and value her spontaneity and easy-going nature, which benefits you far more than her untidy habits damage you. Appreciate that he does laugh, even if it's loud. Appreciate how she juggles so many things at once—work, family, household—and find other ways to manage timely bill mailing.

Why would you do all this? Because it's not only good for

your relationship, it's good for your health. Studies show that when you feel and think appreciation, your heart rate smooths out, good cardiovascular health is supported, your hormonal balance is improved and your immune system enhanced. Your brain functions at full capacity, firing on all cylinders as it were. And the cascade of chemicals and hormones which flow from an appreciative state of mind all benefit the overall well-being of your physical and emotional self.

Collateral benefits. When you look for what works, for what is positive, what you value about your mate and your relationship, not only does your relationship improve dramatically, but your personal health, well-being and likelihood of happy longevity do as well.

29.

Choose Your Thought Reps Wisely

ONE OF MY dogs, Kobe, has epilepsy. It's very well controlled with—of all things—Chinese herbs, but when there's a major stressor, Kobe may be wracked with seizures. In his world, mercifully, there are few major stressors, but one of them is thunder.

We had a major storm in California recently, with a thunderclap in the middle of one afternoon that sounded literally like the sky was falling (no Chicken Little version, this!), crashing down on our very heads.

I rushed over to Kobe and held him, which is about all I can do when he seizes, as my poor puppy trembled all over.

My mind immediately started whirring: "What if he has a major seizure? What if this doesn't stop at trembles and shakes, what if it's a big one, and he's collapsed on the floor, bucking and heaving? He's 15 now, he hasn't had a major seizure in years, what if his heart can't handle it?" And on and on, until I was in almost as bad shape as Kobe.

Then I thought, "What are you doing?" My dog was still trembling and shivering, nothing more, yet I was readying for disaster.

Which is exactly what we do. We rehearse for disaster. We take an event, and rather than address what's actually going on, we let our thoughts tornado through our mind, dragging us into the land of crisis or despair.

The worst of it is, that repetition of thought is what determines how your brain changes and grows. Science these days is teaching us all about neuroplasticity, which simply stated is how the very structure of your brain changes with what you repeatedly think. That how your brain functions then also changes depending on what you think habitually.

If you stay in disaster mode, in "problem" mode, then your brain gets better and better at thinking in that mode, when what we really need, is to be getting better and better at the "appreciation-solution" mode: "What's right with this picture" focus as opposed to the non-appreciative focus of "What's wrong with this picture."

Your thoughts are like the reps you perform to keep your muscles in shape. Whatever reps you do, that's what muscles will grow. If you are to support your brain's development in the direction of happy, healthy longevity, then repeat thoughts of the positive, appreciative, optimistic variety as often as possible.

I stopped my disaster thinking. I shifted into appreciation

mode. I reminded myself that Kobe hadn't had a major seizure in years, that he was a healthy dog despite his age. I reminded myself that I know good vets, that treatments are constantly evolving, that I would always see to it that my beloved pet would get the care he needed. I held him reminding myself that there was nothing more I could do for him in that moment, other than let him feel safe, supported and loved.

It was enough. The trembling eased, all was well. Not just with Kobe, but with myself, as I deliberately reached to grow my brain the way I want it to grow—appreciation and optimism oriented.

Don't let your thoughts mindlessly drag you where you don't want to go. Practice the thoughts that will take you where you *do* want to go. Choose your thought reps wisely!

30.

⚬⚬⚬

Celebrate Your Life With Love on Valentine's Day

DID YOU KNOW there are a gazillion "National Appreciation" days? There's a National Teacher Appreciation Day, National Military Spouse Appreciation Day, an Employee Appreciation Day—all of which are great—as well as a National Squirrel Appreciation Day, even a Cow Appreciation Day ("Go out and give your cow a hug"), but not a single "Appreciate Your Life" day! Yet what could be more important than a day to appreciate all the wonderfulness that makes up your life?

So I have an idea. What if, next Valentine's Day, you chose to fall in love with your *life*! To expand the idea of a day devoted to love beyond that "special person," mate or significant other, and celebrate the love throughout your life: the love of your friends, your pets, your family members, your community, your living space, your occupation, your body, your very self. All the love that permeates your life, if just for a moment, you stop to see it.

Valentine's Day is that moment. Notice, all through your day, the love—the appreciation, the kindness, the caring—that your friends, pets, family, co-workers, cashiers, baristas, all those we share this planet with, extend to us in small and large ways. Smiles, a kind word, a helping hand. These, and so much more, we receive throughout our days. Even more will come your way if you offer *your* love—your smile, your kindness, your help—to those you encounter in the day-in-day-out of your life.

Personally, I make it a practice to say "thank you" when it's unexpected, for things that are too easily taken for granted. I've surprised more than one police officer by saying, "Thank you for keeping us safe," and cleaning personnel in public restrooms by saying, "Thank you for keeping things clean for all of us." You should see the pleased look roadway construction workers give me when I thank them! Or grocery store managers when I ask for "the compliment department." I do my best to keep my awareness high of the many ways in which people, from nears and dears to strangers, fill my life with love.

You see, love isn't only romance and passion. Love is the care with which you do whatever it is you do, the appreciation and respect you give to those you interact with. It is this love, freely and virtually unconsciously given by those I encounter throughout my days, in so many unique and varied ways, that enriches and inspires my life.

Valentine's Day! Yes, of course, celebrate the love with that special someone, but take fullest advantage of this remarkable and wondrous day to appreciate and celebrate the love all around you. Such celebration will not only fill your heart with happiness, but will suffuse your entire body and mind with sweet well-being, precursor to a healthy, happy long life.

31.

Fill Your Life With Happiness: Make It Meaningful

THE ALARM RINGS, you get up, you brush your teeth, you take your shower, you hug your mate, you go to work, you do your job, you get in the car, you pick up the cleaning, you make dinner, you clean up, you go to bed, you kiss your partner good night, you sleep, the alarm rings, you get up, you brush your teeth, you take your shower, you hug your mate… and so it goes.

Then one day you find you can't get out of bed, you can't do it any more, you don't even know why. You're not particularly tired or sick, nothing's wrong between you and your partner—or your out-of-the-nest kids or your friends or your boss—you just know you can't do it any more. All you want to do is lie there and cry.

No, you're not going crazy. Yes, you may be suffering from depression and that possibility needs to be considered, preferably with the help of a trained professional. But in all likelihood, what you are suffering from is a very real and little acknowledged disease of the 21st century: meaninglessness.

Meaninglessness is easy to diagnose. Ask yourself, "What is it all for? The shower, the cleaning, my mate, the job, all of it—why do I do it?" If the answer comes up, "Because I have to" or "Because I should," then you are suffering from meaninglessness. It quite frankly isn't valid, once you're past childhood, to do things because "I have to" or "I should."

One of your greatest freedoms as an adult is the freedom of choice. One of the most powerful choices you can possibly make for yourself, is to choose to do whatever it is that you do with meaning, including those seemingly unimportant daily-dos that add up to a significant portion of your life.

To do something with meaning involves giving that act significance and value. For example, you set your alarm because you care about giving yourself adequate time to get ready for your day. You value yourself too much to rush and slam yourself through your morning. You brush your teeth and take your shower because you value your health, you enjoy feeling well, and you know that cleanliness contributes to good health.

You hug your significant other, not because it's rote, part of the daily drill, but because you want to express to him or her how much you appreciate all the wonderful ways they enhance your life. You go to work and do your job because you enjoy the good feeling of being productive, of being financially responsible for yourself and your family—and so on.

The more you attribute significance and value to the ordinary tasks of everyday life, the more meaning your life acquires, and the more good feelings and happiness you can experience. Even stopping to pick up your spouse's forgotten towel on the floor becomes less an obligation, "I have to, otherwise the house would be a mess," and more a meaningful act, "I want to because I care about making things nice for myself and my family. It's what gives me joy."

A life full of meaning is what leads to life-satisfaction, which in turn contributes significantly to your happy, healthy longevity.

32.

The "Just One" Secret to Fitness (Or Anything Else)

YOU STARE AT the digital read-out on your scale, unbelieving. Ten pounds?! How could you possibly have gained 10 pounds? You eat like a bird! Nothing but fruits and nuts and veggies. Of course there was that pasta dish the other night. And the irresistible danish at work. And the simply sublime butter sauce on the... OK, all right. So you're eating more than just fruits and nuts and veggies. But 10 pounds?!

You swear yourself into your too-tight gym clothes, force yourself through the regimen of machines, spin class and treadmill, and stagger exhausted through the rest of your day.

Get up and do it again the next morning? Ha! No way. Every fiber of your being is screaming for rest. So you rest. A day. Two days. Three—and life takes over, you forget about your solemn promise to yourself to make it to the gym regularly, until you get on the scales again and the 10 pounds have somehow crept up to 12.

A losing battle? No! Just a battle you're taking on as if it were a full scale war.

Switch your focus! Those pounds didn't get there all in a clump. They eased their way into your body. The simplest and most effective way to get rid of them, is to ease them out. To focus on one small thing you *can* do, rather than attempt so much you dump into "can't do" forevermore.

It's the "just one" secret to fitness, that my best friend, a Pilates teacher and studio-owner, shared with me when I despaired of ever getting the knee I had trashed hiking down a mountain back to normal. "Just one leg lift," she said, "You can do one. In a couple of days, do two. Next week, try three." She was right. I could—and did!

Your turn. You want to appreciate those pounds off? Today, do just one sit-up. Right there, on your bedroom floor. No need to get all revved up and into the gym. Not yet. Just do one sit-up. There, done. Or if one sit-up feels too light-weight, do one set of sit-ups, like eight or ten of them. That's it. No more. Just one set.

Tomorrow, repeat. One sit-up, or one set of sit-ups. Don't let yourself do more.

The day after tomorrow, repeat.

On the fourth day, add one more sit-up. If you've been doing one set, add just one more single sit-up. Repeat for the next two days.

Now you're ready for three sit-ups, or one set plus three. Repeat for the next two days.

Every three days, add "just one" to your regimen. Or, add just one new thing to your regimen. Repeat for two more days. And so on.

What you'll find is that it's very easy to do just one exercise, get used to that, and then add one more. Suddenly exercising isn't a big deal. It's quick and easy. You do it regularly, which is far more beneficial to your body and far more effective in achieving weight loss, than slamming yourself into vigorous activity and then doing nothing for a couple of weeks or months.

Within a surprisingly short amount of time, you'll work yourself up to a regimen that suits you and that you can stick with. You won't lose those pounds all at once, but they will come off and stay off.

It doesn't matter whether the exercise you choose is "just one walk around the block" or "just one minute of aerobics" or "just one salsa dance across the living room floor." The "just one" principle allows your body and mind to adjust to increased physical activity gently and efficiently, without the stress that would undo all the health benefits you're trying so valiantly to achieve.

Now, here's the "or anything else" part. No matter what new habit or process you're trying to make part of your routine, whether it's taking time for meditation, reading inspirational books, doing affirmations, or starting a savings account—all of which are great for your happy, healthy long life—adopting the "just one" principle works wonders:

- just one minute of meditation today, maybe just one minute a day for the whole week, then just one minute more the following week,

- just one paragraph of inspirational reading today, maybe just one new paragraph a day for the whole week, then just one more paragraph—so two paragraphs a day for a week,

- just one affirmation today, maybe just the same affirmation every day for the whole week, then add just one more affirmation the following week,

- just one $10 bill into your savings account this week, maybe just $10 a week for the next month—or two or three months, then maybe add just one more dollar, so you're up to $11 per week,

And so on.

Try it! In whatever area of your life you want greater happiness. Switch your focus to what you *can* do, today—and then tomorrow and tomorrow—and enjoy the fruits of your success, now and in your many years to come.

33.

Appreciate Your Obnoxious Crazy Relatives? Sure! Why Not?

YOU LOVE YOUR extended family, you really do. The thought of all those aunts and uncles, in-laws and parents, cousins and various spouses and children warms your heart.

Until it's time for them to descend on your home for a holiday. Be it the 4th of July, Labor Day or Thanksgiving—here they come!

Even if it's just a parent or solitary in-law or wayward cousin, having to deal with relatives you see but once or twice a year can be a trial. It seems so much easier to love them at a distance!

At a distance, you forget all about Aunt Ethel's obnoxious eating habits, or your mother's critical comments about you, your hairdo, your children, your home, your job, your pets, your cooking, your—well, everything.

You welcome them with love and smiles into your home for the feast you've prepared to the very best of your culinary ability, with care for each of their individual preferences, trying not to let your frantic last-minute running around show.

Here they are and here's the feast. All is well.

But it doesn't take long for Aunt Ethel's chomping to get at you, or those critical comments to make you grit your teeth (biting back the sharp retort you long to give), nor for you to think unkind thoughts of your cousin's new wife (a plunging neckline and leather micro-skirt? At the family Labor Day barbeque?).

Time for a shift! A shift in focus, that is. The more you allow yourself to notice your relatives' irritating behaviors, the more unhappy you will become. The more unhappy you become, the more likely that you'll end up with a headache and a pissy attitude, causing yourself unnecessary stress which does nothing good for your immune system or your long-term well-being.

Shift. Think about how much Aunt Ethel loves her food. The food you so lovingly prepared. So she has horrible table manners, so? She's having a good time, thanks to you.

Your mother's critical take on the world is her problem. You like yourself as you are, along with your hairdo, your children, your home, your job, your pets, your whatever else she's poking at. Criticism is often a misguided attempt to improve things for others so they can be happier. This is just your mother's way of loving you. Weird, I know, but again—not your problem. Let the critical comments flow off you like water off a duck's back. Irrelevant, no different than bad late-night talk show yada-yada. Just filler. Unimportant.

So the new wife is showing off her stuff? Who cares? It makes her happy, and certainly doesn't mean you have to imitate her style.

Focus on what does matter, on what you can appreciate: the guests who are enjoying themselves, how nicely your casserole turned out, that the table looks lovely. Focus on how grateful you are to have a family—of one, or two, or many. Focus on how good it is to be alive, and value all the good things in your life. Focus on appreciating and being grateful, let the rest just roll on by, and even your crazy obnoxious relatives won't seem so bad.

Such is the stuff of which happy, healthy longevity is made.

34.

Will Boredom Steal Your Love Away?

YOU LOOK OVER at the love of your life, head shoved under the sink, patiently repairing that drip-drip-drip that's been driving you nuts. You sigh as you put away the dish you've just dried, pick up the next one. Is this all there is? Is marriage just one long series of chores, errands, and work to be done? Oh sure, you have some laughs and nice times together, but what happened to the excitement? The passion? The "I-can't-wait-to-see-you" flutter? Your guy is a good man, you don't want to trade him in for a newer, zippier model, but oh, how you are bored!! Your mind drifts away to a novel thought—an affair?

What you don't know is the love of your life, as he replaces the drain trap and tightens the hose clamp, is thinking roughly the same thing. He loves you, he's comfortable with you, you have some laughs and nice times, but what happened to the closeness? That feeling of intense involvement, when your life together was interesting, even exciting? There's only so much joy he can drum up over watching the tube together. Heck, he's having more passion coaching the grandkids at Little League! It hits him with discouraging certainty, even as he hits his head on a pipe, he's bored!! His mind drifts to—an affair?

Boredom. A stealth bomb destroying the passion, the engagement, the closeness that makes for true happiness in your marriage, your relationship. It creeps up on you without your hardly noticing until—blam! There you are, thinking the unthinkable. An affair.

A study of 123 married couples seven years into their marriage, and then again, nine years later, 16 years into their marriage, showed that boredom does indeed reduce closeness between the spouses. This reduced closeness is what in turn causes reduced satisfaction with the relationship (*Psychological Science*, April 14, 2009).

How do you alleviate boredom? By appreciating each other, by valuing each other as you did during your courtship. By bringing more meaning into your time together, making that time genuine "quality time" as opposed to wondering what you might have to talk about.

Here are five ways to do just that:

1. Turn "Date Night" Into More Than Dinner-and-a-Movie

Just because you're married or in a long term relationship doesn't mean you should stop dating! Many couples know how to make one night of the week or weekend a "date night." Take "date night" one step further, so it doesn't turn into same-old, same-old. Be innovative. Take turns surprising each other with where you go or what you do on your date.

Deliberately come up with ideas that let you experience new things together. Anything from exploring the night sky at the local observatory, to hitting the state fair, to trying foods from exotic lands. Exploring new things together is one of the ways you learn new things about each other, things that make you go, "Wow, you're pretty terrific!" all over again.

2. Take Up a Hobby Together

Find something new and different you'd really like to do together, whether it's kite-flying, glass-blowing or collecting stamps. Make regular time every week to do that thing together. Make it matter! Be excited and passionate about it, talk about it, look forward to it.

3. Get a Question Book

You may think you know everything there is to know about your sweetheart after so many years. Not! People grow and change throughout their lives. When you lose interest in finding out what makes him or her tick, they may lose interest in you. There are wonderful books filled with lists of questions you can ask your mate—some thought provoking, some silly, some just plain fun—all of which generate more to love and appreciate about him or her.

34.

4. Play Word/Board Games Together

Watching TV together is fun, but it isn't exactly couple-interactive. Make an effort to click off the tube and dive into a word/board game, just the two of you. Whether it's scrabble, or putting a puzzle together, or a "trivia for 2" game, playing together can enhance your appreciation of each other, which in turn helps to keep your love strong.

5. Volunteer Together

Volunteering has wonderful benefits, it gives you a sense of purpose and accomplishment. In addition, studies show volunteering is good for your health. When you volunteer together and work side by side for the benefit of your community, church, neighborhood or favorite cause, you share that sense of purpose and accomplishment. It brings you closer.

There you go. Five easy ways to banish boredom from your marriage without a fatal plunge into an affair or other diversion (gambling, alcohol, excessive shopping) detrimental to your relationship, plus the undeniable health, happiness, and longevity benefits of a fun, close, loving relationship.

35.

Anger: Release First, Appreciate Second

YOU'RE HAVING A lousy day at work. Your boss is entirely unreasonable, expecting you to be in three places at once, and when you do exactly what he asked you to, he bawls you out. When you try (biting your tongue very hard so as not to scream) to gently (!) point out that you were only following his directives, you get yelled at even louder!

At this point there is nothing you would like better than to grab your boss by the throat and throw him bodily out the window. You'd even settle for just telling him off, as long as you could do it at top volume. But no, that little voice within you kicks in, "This is your boss, he could fire you and then where would you be?" You just sigh, squashing all those feelings.

Then when you get home and your significant other forgot to get take-out, again all you want to do is rant, but then here comes that little voice, "You can't do that! You're a good person. So your partner forgot dinner, what's the big deal? Besides if you yell, maybe he or she won't love you anymore, and maybe you aren't that good person you think you are, maybe you're really just a horrible angry abusive person." You sigh, squashing all those feelings.

As saintly as it might seem, squashing angry feelings may end up killing you. There is a high correspondence between stuffed angry feelings, resentment and cancer. Stuffing feelings can also lead to heart attacks, ulcers, and various other equally unpleasant conditions.

However, as you are only too aware, dumping anger all over people is highly inappropriate. Dealing with your anger, however, is not only appropriate but necessary, if you're not to develop rage, resentment, and a subsequent array of self-destructive behaviors. Dealing with your anger consists of releasing that anger in a safe manner, and then switching your focus to what you can value and appreciate in the situation that would help you to resolve it.

1. Release Your Anger

Releasing your anger safely can be easily and effectively done by, for example, writing your feelings in the form of a letter *you never send*, or writing your feelings in your private journal, or beating the you-know out of a pillow safely placed in the middle of your bed (a pillow you name boss/significant other or whoever). Do whichever method you choose until you feel the anger dissipate.

You always have the additional option of consulting a

mental health professional or pastoral counselor if you find releasing the anger on your own problematic. But release you must, for you'll never be able to genuinely appreciate and move on if anger is still stuck in your craw.

2. Appreciate

Now that you've released the anger, figure out what really matters to you in the situation, what would be of value to you. If with your boss, it's to do a good job, go for that: "Boss, I'm confused. I want to do a good job for you, but I'm unclear as to what you want done first. Please tell me." Then write down whatever boss says, in front of him, so there's no confusion on his part later on.

If with your significant other, it's to make sure dinner gets handled, and, if one of you forgets that it was "your night," then have a discussion about that: "Hon, what do you think would be a good fallback plan if the usual dinner arrangement doesn't happen?" If you agree that whoever forgot (or got too busy, or whatever) takes the other out or orders in Chinese, great. There's no reason to get mad when you already know dinner is handled one way or the other.

The less you allow anger to take over, the better. There are few situations in life that are worth the strain anger puts on your future well-being, and by extension, on your longevity.

36.

Ditch the "Have-To's" and Get to the (Way More Fun) "Want-To's"

EVER NOTICE THE list of "have-to's" you've got going? As in "have-to" get up and get yourself going, "have-to" get everybody fed-dressed-out-the-door, "have-to" get to work, "have-to" do the work, "have-to" put up with a boss/co-worker/client you can't stand, "have-to" run errands, do chores, pay bills, and on and on.

When life is reduced to a list of "have-to's," it becomes drudgery, just a long list of dutiful things you must do as a responsible adult. Over time, the toll on your immune system, your cardiovascular system and your nervous system is significant, much to the detriment of your current and future well-being.

What happened?! Growing up was supposed to be fun. Yeah, right. No big surprise that your daydreams are all of lying on a beach somewhere, with absolutely no "have-to's" whatsoever, other people being responsible for meeting your every desire and whim thank-you-very-much.

But what if you could transform being responsible into being response-able? Not in the form of some clever word-play that really doesn't change anything, but into a meaningful change with substance.

What if you could transform "I have to" into "I want to"? Such that you would *want* to get yourself up and going, *want* to get everybody fed-dressed-out-the-door, *want* to get to work, *want* to do the work, *want* to figure out how to work with a boss/co-worker/client you can't stand, *want* to run the errands, do the chores, pay the bills, and on and on.

All it takes is thinking for a moment about what you are trying to accomplish with your "have-to." For example, you "have-to" get yourself up and going in the morning. Why? What are you trying to accomplish? You want to have a productive and good day. Ah! So you do value the end result. Focus on that.

Or, you "have-to" put up with a boss/co-worker/client you can't stand. Again, ask yourself, why? What are you trying to accomplish? You want to do a good job so you can get a raise, a bonus, or a promotion. There you go—that's your end result. Something you can genuinely value and appreciate. Focus on that.

Don't sit there bemoaning how awful it is that you

"have-to" put up with these folks, instead, focus on the good-feels a raise or promotion will give you.

The principle is the same regardless of what your particular "have-to" (or unending list of "have-to's") is! Take a step back and ask yourself, "What am I looking to accomplish here? What good/fun/rewarding result do I want to have happen by doing this "have-to"?"

Then take your focus off the seeming drudgery of the "have-to" and put it where it belongs. On the much anticipated, greatly appreciated, joy of your success with whatever it is.

Now you've become genuinely response-able. Able to respond to the situation in a way that brings you happiness: a sure-fire path to happy, healthy longevity.

37.

Women Complain, Men Leave

YOU'RE ROLLING YOUR cart down the supermarket aisle, when you bump into (literally) your friend whom you haven't seen in—well, awhile. She asks, "Where's your husband?" and you say, "Oh, I dunno. Probably doing something around the house." Your friend laughs and says, "Well, I knew it couldn't last. The two of you doing everything together." That stings. Because you remember all those years when you and your mate used to do pretty much everything together, from groceries to chores to laundry to workouts. Now it seems you do everything separately. You don't remember when or how that happened.

As you think about it, you realize you spend a lot less time together, and what time you do spend together is all about the "business" of a relationship. What's the schedule, should we buy this or forego that, did you/he remember to do yet another on that unending list of chores, which friends are next on the "must get together" list and so on. The intimacy has diminished in your love-life; not that you love each other any less, but that closeness, that feeling of true connection has faded.

You've complained about the lack of closeness, of course you have! You've complained to your sister, your girlfriends, your co-workers, your mani-pedi gal, all of whom sympathize greatly. You've complained and nagged about it to your spouse, but that only seems to drive him further away.

And there you have it. Women complain, men leave.

Oh, they don't necessarily leave physically, but whereas women speak up loudly in relationships about what's wrong, what's bothering them, men respond more often than not by simply leaving. First emotionally, then mentally, lastly physically.

Men are trained by our culture and society not to whine, not to complain, to be stoic and put up with hardship. They bring that attitude into their relationships as well. Which is why a wife is often surprised to find her mate has strayed. She assumed that since he wasn't complaining, all was well.

Not! What to do? Pay as much attention to the connection side of your relationship as you do to the business side. Openly express your appreciation to your mate, let him or her know how valuable they are—to you, to your family, to the world—every day. Purposefully join in those activities he enjoys, be that the ballgame on Sunday afternoon, his new interest in golf, or his fascination with that software program.

Openly, deliberately, value what matters to him. If you

can't join in, be supportive. Be interested and enthusiastic. Let him know how much you appreciate the pleasure these activities bring to your mate. Be engaged in his work, show interest in what makes up his day and engage him in yours.

You'll be contributing mightily not just to your increased closeness, but also to your mutual well-being and that long happy life together so dear to the both of you.

38.

꼭꼭꼭

Don't Leave Yourself Out of Thanksgiving Gratitude

WHETHER IT'S FEBRUARY, April or July, Thanksgiving will be upon us before we know it, that time of year when "Get your gratitude on!" is the theme of the day (along with football and turkey). And indeed, you will have your gratitude well in gear.

You are ready to express your gratefulness for your family, your friends, your job (maybe, could be a stretch), Pilates, football, the roof over your head, your pets, your new tablet, the Macy's sale, and lots more.

The only thing notably lacking in your list of "Things I am grateful for" is *you*! Ah yes. Can we talk? Because when it comes to you, yourself, your list is composed of: "I'm too fat, too thin, too tall, too short, not smart enough, not getting it together enough, too lazy, too ambitious, too talkative, too quiet, fashion-challenged, a procrastinator," and that's the short list. The rest would take up several more pages.

Yet you are, with all your supposed lacks, the most astonishing combination of flesh, blood, bone and consciousness ever to grace the earth.

I invite you to be grateful, at Thanksgiving or any other time—for *you*.

Not in some overblown narcissistic way, "I'm grateful for me because I'm so much better than all you other humans out there," but with the graciousness available to us all: "I'm grateful for all that I am and am becoming." There's humility in that statement, a simple recognition that how you are right now is truly OK, and that the future holds the possibility of yet more of whatever you want to be.

Make your list of all that you appreciate about yourself. It may take you a while if you're not used to this exercise, but it's well worth the effort in terms of the value-add to your long term well-being and future happiness, I promise.

I'll share with you some of my list, to give you an example: I'm grateful that I'm pretty darn healthy most of the time, that I manage to keep my wits about me for the most part, that sometimes people think I'm funny. I'm grateful that I have ears to hear the sound of wind in the trees, of laughter, of music, that I have eyes to see the splendors of our natural world, a heart that quickens to kindness and gets sad when I witness or experience despair. There's more, but you get the gist.

When you reflect on what there is about yourself that you appreciate and are grateful for, you'll find that you have so much to be happy about, and to share with others. It is an odd truism that only self-love allows us to truly love others. Honest self-gratitude, without arrogance or strut, allows us to be grateful for others with whom we share this amazing planet, to be optimistic about their future as well as ours.

LAST WORDS

THERE YOU HAVE it. An assortment of tips, tools and techniques for how to use appreciation in your everyday life, so that you can enjoy a happy, healthy long life, a life truly worth living. What I wish ardently for you.

In addition, there are innumerable resources on the Web, specifically devoted to helping you increase your gratitude and happiness. You'll find some in the "Resources" section of this book.

A bumper sticker I saw sums up how to achieve happy, healthy longevity better than anything else I could possibly say:

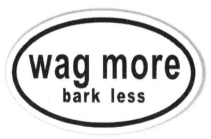

REFERENCES

Chapter One

1. https://www.census.gov/prod/cen2010/briefs/
   c2010br-09.pdf

2. https://youtu.be/Cx5KaA3Be0E

3. phyllissues.com/

4. Aashmita Nayar, "The Final Photoshoot: Yoga Guru BKS
   Iyengar Performing Yoga At The Age Of 95," *HuffPost India*, June 21, 2015.

5. http://widerimage.reuters.com/story/
   california-seniors-police-patrol

6. https://www.census.gov/prod/cen2010/briefs/
   c2010br-09.pdf

7. http://www.nydailynews.com/life-style/health/

new-jersey-woman-astrid-thoenig-celebrates-100th-birth-day-heading-work-article-1.403954

8. https://www.youtube.com/watch?v=O8wr3wLAjwk

9. https://www.cardealexpert.com/fyi/margaret-dunning/

10. https://en.wikipedia.org/wiki/Margaret_Dunning

11. http://www.adlercentenarians.org/cent_spotlight.htm

12. http://www.foxnews.com/us/2015/06/06/100-year-old-dressmaker-finishes-1051st-dress-for-african-children/

13. http://www.adlercentenarians.org/cent_spotlight.htm

14. Richard Corliss and Michael D. Lemonick, "How to Live to Be 100," *Time*, August 30, 2004.

15. "Legends of Longevity," *Time,* June 8, 2015.

Chapter Two

1. Deepak Chopra, *Ageless Body, Timeless Mind.* New York: Harmony Books, 1993, p. 17.

2. J. C. Barefoot, W. G. Dahlstrom, and R. B. Williams, Jr., "Hostility, CHD Incidence, and Total Mortality: A 25-Year Follow-Up Study of 255 Physicians," *Psychosomatic Medicine*, 45, 1 (1983), pp. 59–63.

3. Ellen J. Langer, *Counter Clockwise.* New York: Ballantine Books, 2009.

4. I. C. Siegler, P. T. Costa, B. H. Brummett, et al., "Patterns of Change in Hostility from College to Midlife

in the UNC Alumni Heart Study Predict High-Risk Status," *Psychosomatic Medicine*, 65, 5 (2003), pp. 738–745.

5. D. M. Becker, L. R. Yanek, T. F. Moy, et al., "General Well-Being Is Strongly Protective Against Future Coronary Heart Disease Events in an Apparently Healthy High-Risk Population," Abstract #103966, presented at *American Heart Association Scientific Sessions*, Anaheim, CA, November 12, 2001.

Chapter Three

1. http://www.eurekalert.org/pub_releases/2015-06/ps-kca_1060915.php

2. http://articles.mercola.com/sites/articles/archive/2010/02/04/stress-linked-to-cancer.aspx

3. Doc Childre and Howard Martin, *The HeartMath Solution*. San Francisco: Harper, 1999, pp. 37, 40.

4. Ibid.

5. Noelle Nelson and Jeannine LeMare Calaba, *The Power of Appreciation*. Hillsboro, Oregon: Beyond Words, 2003, pp. 11-13.

6. Ibid.

Chapter Four

1. "Positive Emotions in Early Life and Longevity: Findings from the Nun Study" conducted by Deborah D. Danner and David A. Snowdon, along with Wallace V. Friesen and researchers at the College of Medicine at the University of Kentucky, 2001.

2. http://www.huffingtonpost.com/2011/11/01/happiness-long-life-_n_1068209.html

3. http://www.pnas.org/content/108/45/18244.abstract http://www.webmd.com/women/features/gratitute-health-boost

4. http://longevity.about.com/od/inyour20s30sand40s/fl/The-Health-Benefits-of-Gratitude.htm

5. http://www.ncbi.nlm.nih.gov/pubmed/7484873

6. https://www.templeton.org/grateful

7. http://greatergood.berkeley.edu/pdfs/GratitudePDFs/7McCullough-GratefulDisposition.pdf

8. http://pss.sagepub.com/content/early/2015/06/02/0956797615581491.abstract

9. http://www.webmd.com/women/features/gratitute-health-boost

10. Martin E.P. Seligman, *Learned Optimism*. New York: Pocket Books, 1990.

11. http://www.cbsnews.com/news/study-optimists-live-longer/

12. http://bit.ly/1Kb4k8Y

13. http://www.cdc.gov/heartdisease/statistics.htm

14. Albert Rosenfeld, *Prolongevity II*. New York: Alfred A. Knopf, 1985.

15. Stephen P. Jewett, "Longevity and the Longevity Syndrome," *The Gerontologist*, 13, 1 (1973), pp. 91-99.

16. Charles J. Pellerin, *How NASA Builds Teams: Mission Critical Soft Skills for Scientists, Engineers, and Project Teams*, New York: Wiley, 2009, p. 157.

Chapter Five

1. A. J. Crum and E. J. Langer, "Mind-Set Matters: Exercise and the Placebo Effect," *Psychological Science*, 18, 2 (2007), pp. 165-171.

2. http://bit.ly/1RCd3oE

Chapter Six

1. https://www.nwba.org/about/general-information/history/

2. http://www.amp1basketball.com/

3. https://en.wikipedia.org/wiki/Beck_Weathers

4. http://www.scientificamerican.com/article/stephen-hawking-als/
   https://en.wikipedia.org/wiki/Stephen_Hawking

5. http://www.csmonitor.com/1997/0811/081197.feat.feat.2.html

6. https://en.wikipedia.org/wiki/Joey_Moss

7. http://news.yahoo.com/video/92-old-woman-breaks-marathon-144634211-cbs.html
http://fox40.com/2015/06/01/92-year-old-becomes-oldest-woman-to-complete-marathon/

8. Deepak Chopra, *Ageless Body, Timeless Mind.* New York: Harmony Books, 1993, p. 248.

9. http://www.nytimes.com/1994/06/23/us/study-finds-that-weight-training-can-benefit-the-very-old.html

10. M. Fiatarone, E. Marks, N. Ryan, C. Meredith, L. Lipsitz, & W. Evans, "High-intensity strength training in nonagenarians," *Journal of the American Medical Association*, 263, 22 (1990), pp. 3029-3034.

11. B. R. Levy, M. D. Slade, S. R. Kunkel, et al., "Longevity Increased by Positive Self-Perceptions of Aging," *Journal of Personality and Social Psychology*, 83, 2 (2002), pp. 261-270.

12. Lisa Schwarzbaum, "Fashion's Hot New Age," *Time*, April 20, 2015.

13. https://en.wikipedia.org/wiki/John_Glenn

14. https://youtu.be/FIMd5KFG1vQ
https://youtu.be/2BcCdiC-91s
https://www.youtube.com/watch?v=hjHnWz3EyHs
https://youtu.be/jAZLDKw7MeQ

15. http://psr.sagepub.com/content/19/3/235

16. http://www.nature.com/ng/journal/v47/n7/full/ng.3285.html

17. Dawson Church, *The Genie in Your Genes: Epigenetic Medicine and the New Biology of Intention.* Santa Rosa, California: Elite Books, 2007, p. 32.

18. http://www.sciencedirect.com/science/article/pii/S0092656614000956

RESOURCES

3 Good Things

http://www.3bonneschoses.com/home/

A gratitude journal app that remembers every nice thing you write in it. A new way to never forget even the littlest moments of happiness in your life.

Happify.com

www.happify.com

Build skills for lasting happiness: *Happify* turns the latest innovations in the science of happiness into activities and games that help you lead a more fulfilling life.

Huffington Post/Happiness

http://www.huffingtonpost.com/news/happiness/

Includes blogs, news and community conversations about happiness.

Huffington Post/Good News

http://www.huffingtonpost.com/good-news/

A spotlight on what's inspiring and positive.

Daily Hooplaha

http://hooplaha.com/

Sure to make you smile with stories of happiness and gratitude.

Gratefulness

http://www.gratefulness.org/

Deepen your gratitude awareness with these daily practices.

Gratitude Quotes

http://www.brainyquote.com/quotes/keywords/gratitude.html

Insightful quotes to uplift you anytime.

Louie Schwartzberg: Nature. Beauty. Gratitude.

https://www.ted.com/talks/
louie_schwartzberg_nature_beauty_gratitude?language=en

Louie Schwartzberg's stunning time-lapse photography accompanied by powerful words from Benedictine monk

Brother David Steindl-Rast. Serves as a meditation on being grateful for every day.

60 Minutes: Living to 90 and Beyond

http://www.cbsnews.com/news/living-to-90-and-beyond/

Even though this series of interviews with 90+ folks centers on the physical aspects of their longevity and makes no mention of psychological or emotional components, it's well worth checking out.

ABOUT THE AUTHOR

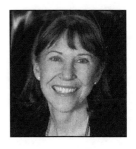

NOELLE C. NELSON, PhD, psychologist, consultant and international speaker, has authored 14 books, among which *Your Man Is Wonderful, Dangerous Relationships,* and *Make More Money by Making Your Employees Happy.* All of Dr. Nelson's work focuses on empowering individuals to be happier, healthier, and more successful in their personal lives, at work, at home and in relationships.

Dr. Nelson is also a regular contributor to HitchedMag.com and The Huffington Post.

Dr. Nelson holds advanced degrees in clinical psychology from the United States International University, and sociology degrees from the University of California at Los Angeles and the Sorbonne, Paris. She is a licensed clinical psychologist.

For more tips on how to benefit from appreciation, gratitude and happiness in your life, visit Dr. Nelson at:

Website
www.noellenelson.com
Facebook
www.facebook.com/Dr.NoelleNelson
Twitter
@drnoellenelson.com

Made in the USA
San Bernardino, CA
07 December 2015